AF566772

Anti-VEGF

Developments in Ophthalmology

Vol. 46

Anti-VEGF

Volume Editors

F. Bandello Milan
M. Battaglia Parodi Milan

Co-Editors

A.J. Augustin Karlsruhe
P. Iacono Rome
R.O. Schlingemann Amsterdam
U. Schmidt-Erfurth Vienna
F.D. Verbraak Amsterdam

12 figures, 5 in color, and 13 tables, 2010

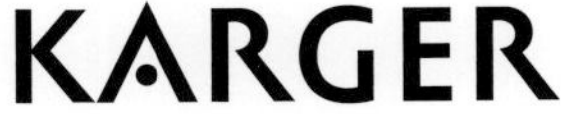

Basel · Freiburg · Paris · London · New York · Bangalore · Bangkok · Shanghai · Singapore · Tokyo · Sydney

Francesco Bandello
Department of Ophthalmology
University Vita-Salute Scientific Institute
San Raffaele
Via Olgettina, 60
IT–20132 Milano (Italy)

Maurizio Battaglia Parodi
Department of Ophthalmology
University Vita-Salute Scientific Institute
San Raffaele
Via Olgettina, 60
IT–20132 Milano (Italy)

Library of Congress Cataloging-in-Publication Data

Anti-VEGF / volume editors, Francesco Bandello, M. Battaglia Parodi ; co-editors, A. Augustin ... [et al.].
p. ; cm. -- (Developments in ophthalmology, ISSN 0250-3751 ; v. 46)
Includes bibliographical references and indexes.
ISBN 978-3-8055-9529-2 (hard cover : alk. paper) -- ISBN 978-3-8055-9530-8 (e-ISBN)
1. Eye--Blood-vessels--Diseases--Chemotherapy. 2. Vascular endothelial growth factors--Antagonists--Therapeutic use. I. Bandello, F. (Francesco) II. Battaglia Parodi, M. (Maurizio) III. Series: Developments in ophthalmology ; v. 46. 0250-3751
[DNLM: 1. Eye Diseases--therapy. 2. Vascular Endothelial Growth Factors--therapeutic use. 3. Neovascularization, Pathologic--therapy. W1 DE998NG v.46 2010 / WW 166 A6334 2010]
RE720.A58 2010
617.7′061--dc22

2010025184

Bibliographic Indices. This publication is listed in bibliographic services, including Current Contents® and Index Medicus.

www.karger.com
Printed in Switzerland on acid-free and non-aging paper (ISO 9706) by Reinhardt Druck, Basel
ISSN 0250–3751
ISBN 978–3–8055–9529–2
e-ISBN 978–3–8055–9530–8

Contents

List of Contributors

A.J. Augustin, Prof.
Augenklinik
Moltkestrasse 90
DE–76133 Karlsruhe (Germany)
E-Mail albertjaugustin@googlemail.com

F. Bandello, Prof.
Department of Ophthalmology
University Vita-Salute Scientific Institute
San Raffaele
Via Olgettina, 60
IT–20132 Milano (Italy)
E-Mail bandello.francesco@hsr.it

M. Battaglia Parodi, Dr.
Department of Ophthalmology
University Vita-Salute Scientific Institute
San Raffaele
Via Olgettina, 60
IT–20132 Milano (Italy)
E-Mail battagliaparodi.maurizio@hsr.it

M. Bolz, Dr.
Department of Ophthalmology and
Optometry
Medical University Vienna
Waehringer Guertel 18-20
AT–1090 Vienna (Austria)
E-Mail matthias.bolz@meduniwien.ac.at

A. Buchholz, Dr.
Augenklinik
Moltkestrasse 90
DE–76133 Karlsruhe (Germany)
E-Mail Andreas.Buchholz@
klinikum-karlsruhe.de

P. Buchholz, Dr.
Augenklinik
Moltkestrasse 90
DE–76133 Karlsruhe (Germany)
E-Mail apkbuchholz@yahoo.de

W. Buehl, Dr.
Department of Ophthalmology and
Optometry
Medical University Vienna
Waehringer Guertel 18-20
AT–1090 Vienna (Austria)
E-Mail wolf.buehl@meduniwien.ac.at

H. de Groot, Dr.
Augenklinik
Moltkestrasse 90
DE–76133 Karlsruhe (Germany)
E-Mail developments@dr-de-groot.de

P. Iacono, Dr.
Fondazione G.B. Bietti per l'Oftalmologia
IRCCS (Istituto di Ricovero e Cura a
Carattere Scientifico)
Via Livenza 3
IT–00198 Rome (Italy)
E-Mail pierluigi.iacono@libero.it

M.J. Jager, Prof.
Department of Ophthalmology
LUMC
PO Box 9600
NL–2300 RC Leiden (The Netherlands)
E-Mail m.j.jager@lumc.nl

J. Kirchhof, Dr.
Augenklinik
Moltkestrasse 90
DE–76133 Karlsruhe (Germany)
E-Mail jannakirchhof@googlemail.com

G.S. Missotten, Prof.
Department Ophthalmology
Academic Medical Center
Meibergdreef 9
NL–1100DD Amsterdam (The Netherlands)
E-Mail guy.missotten@uzleuven.be

C. Mitsch, Dr.
Department of Ophthalmology and Optometry
Medical University Vienna
Waehringer Guertel 18-20
AT–1090 Vienna (Austria)
E-Mail christoph.mitsch@meduniwien.ac.at

A. Pollreisz, Dr.
Department of Ophthalmology and Optometry
Medical University Vienna
Waehringer Guertel 18-20
AT–1090 Vienna (Austria)
E-Mail andreas.pollreisz@meduniwien.ac.at

S. Sacu, Dr.
Department of Ophthalmology and Optometry
Medical University Vienna
Waehringer Guertel 18-20
AT–1090 Vienna (Austria)
E-Mail stefan.sacu@meduniwien.ac.at

R.O. Schlingemann, Prof.
Medical Retina Unit and Ocular Angiogenesis Group
Department of Ophthalmology
Academic Medical Center
University of Amsterdam, A2-122
NL–1100 DD Amsterdam (The Netherlands)
E-Mail r.schlingemann@amc.uva.nl

U. Schmidt-Erfurth, Prof.
Department of Ophthalmology and Optometry
Medical University Vienna
Waehringer Guertel 18-20
AT–1090 Vienna (Austria)
E-Mail ursula.schmidt-erfurth@meduniwien.ac.at

V. Schmit-Eilenberger, Dr.
Augenklinik
Moltkestrasse 90
DE–76133 Karlsruhe (Germany)
E-Mail dr.schmit-eilenberger@email.de

S. Scholl, Dr.
Augenklinik
Moltkestrasse 90
DE–76133 Karlsruhe (Germany)
E-Mail s-scholl@gmx.de

M.J. Siemerink, Dr.
Medical Retina Unit and Ocular Angiogenesis Group
Department of Ophthalmology
Academic Medical Center
University of Amsterdam, A2-122
NL–1100 DD Amsterdam (The Netherlands)
E-Mail m.j.siemerink@amc.uva.nl

F.D. Verbraak, Dr.
Departments of Ophthalmology and Biomedical Engineering & Physics
Academic Medical Center
Meibergdreef 9
NL–1105 AZ Amsterdam (The Netherlands)
E-Mail f.d.verbraak@amc.nl

Preface

The development of vascular endothelial growth factor inhibitors for the treatment of ocular neovascularization and macular edema can be regarded as the beginning of a new era in ophthalmological therapy. Before the year 2000, the treatment of any vascular abnormality in the macular region was merely restricted to conventional laser photocoagulation. Indubitably, laser treatment represents a destructive procedure which leads to a permanent scar and brings about a retinal sensitivity deterioration in all cases. Since 2000, photodynamic therapy with verteporfin has been introduced as the first attempt to couple laser energy with a light-sensitive drug in an attempt to treat choroidal neovascularization through a relatively non-destructive form of therapy. Nevertheless, photodynamic therapy can provide only a very limited visual acuity improvement, especially in choroidal neovascularization secondary to age-related macular degeneration and pathologic myopia.

In an attempt to improve the functional outcomes, many researchers have studied the potential application of anti-angiogenic agents on ocular diseases. Previous investigations have demonstrated that vascular endothelial growth factor plays an important role in promoting angiogenesis and vascular leakage in several ocular pathologic conditions. The main goals of antivascular endothelial growth factor therapy are the inhibition of growth and development of new vessels, along with the reduction of vascular permeability.

The encouraging results of the most important randomized clinical trials regarding the efficacy of ranibizumab and pegaptanib on subfoveal choroidal neovascularization in relation to age-related macular degeneration have greatly influenced current medical practice. As a result, in the last few years, many applications have been proposed in an effort to treat several vascular diseases of the eye.

This aim of this book is to help update residents, general ophthalmologists, and retina specialists on the latest applications of antivascular endothelial growth factor therapy in ocular diseases. After an outline of the treatment principles, it covers a large number of topics, including age-related macular degeneration, pathologic myopia, angioid streaks, inflammatory diseases, hereditary dystrophies, retinal vein occlusions, diabetic retinopathy, ocular tumors, and anterior segment neovascularizations. We hope that each chapter will stimulate the interest of readers working in this field.

Francesco Bandello, Milan

Bandello F, Battaglia Parodi M (eds): Anti-VEGF.
Dev Ophthalmol. Basel, Karger, 2010, vol 46, pp 1–3

Angiostatic and Angiogenic Factors

Heink de Groot · Vera Schmit-Eilenberger · Janna Kirchhof · Albert J. Augustin

Augenklinik, Karlsruhe, Germany

Abstract

Both diminution of angiostatic and increment of angiogenic factors seem to contribute to neovascularization in the eye under pathologic conditions. They are presented here separately. The involved proteins can change their role during the process of neovascularization from promoters to inhibitors and vice versa. Angiostatic factors can be divided into passive, active, unspecific and specific ones. Some of them act during neovascularization as members of feedback loops by modifying the effects of their angiogenic counterparts. Among the angiogenic factors VEGF is the most important. Nevertheless other stimulating proteins exist in large numbers. Together with their static counterparts they form a complex network which controls neovascularization under physiologic as well as pathologic conditions.

A short introduction into the topics of angiostatic and angiogenic factors is given. All molecules mentioned and their interactions within the organism will be discussed in the following article.

Angiostatic Factors in the Eye

Under healthy conditions the vascular system of the eye is thought to be stable. Normal angiogenesis is concluded during early childhood and only reappears under certain pathologic conditions. While one common trigger of neovascularization in many eye diseases is ischemia, neovascularization can also occur without significant ischemia. This is the case in wet age-related macular degeneration (AMD). However, hypoxia and/or alterations of the perfusion are still under discussion to be an important cofactor in the pathogenesis of this disease entity.

In ischemic neovascularization, new capillaries typically sprout from branches of the retinal arteries. In contrast, the neovascularization in AMD originates from the choriocapillary layer. The physiological stability of the ocular vascular system is an equilibrium between angiostatic and angiogenic factors. The vasculature is stable as long as the angiostatic factors are ahead. Pathologic conditions such as ischemia or inflammation shift the balance towards angiogenic factors which are released by the damaged cells. On the other hand the unpredictable appearance of neovascularization during dry AMD which cannot be prevented by anti-inflammatory treatment strongly points out that also a loss of angiostatic factors alone can lead to instability of the constructive vascular boundaries of the eye.

The strong angiostasis that is crucial for the function of the eye is maintained by angiostatic factors in every involved tissue starting from the specialized guards of the blood-retinal barrier down to unspecific ingredients of the blood fluid. The angiostatic effect is not only locally distributed but also stepwise during stages of angiogenesis. Due to the defensive nature of static concepts, not only active components such as inhibitor proteins but also passive stabilizing members of the extracellular matrix can be accounted to the angiostatic system.

Thus, collagens, elastins and fibrin constitute a first barrier for angiogenesis. These molecules have to be actively degraded and the respective proteases are controlled by protease inhibitors. Tissue inhibitors of metalloproteinases are specific metalloproteinase inhibitors while the serum component α_2-macroglobulin unspecifically inhibits metalloproteinases. Another protein that interferes with pericellular proteolysis required for migration and proliferation of endothelial cells is thrombospondin which is present in platelet granules and is released following platelet activation. If proteolytic degradation of capillary basement membranes occurs, a fragment of the collagen type 18 called endostatin is released. It specifically inhibits proliferation of endothelial cells and angiogenesis.

Other passive components of vascular stability are the VE cadherins that are involved in intercellular tight junctions – the constituting basis of the blood-retinal barrier. VE cadherins are members of a large family of adhesion proteins called cadherins that build intercellular contacts like desmosomes throughout the body. VE cadherins have to be degraded before angiogenesis can occur. Their degradation is triggered by vascular endothelial growth factors (VEGF) via the VEGFR-2 receptor.

More active components of vascular structural stability of the eye are proteins that are secreted by the cells of the blood-retinal barrier. A protein that maintains stability after maturation of newly grown capillaries is angiopoietin-1. It is produced by pericytes. Its presence in mature capillaries improves continuity of the basal membranes and the adherence of pericytes to endothelial cells. During angiogenesis it promotes capillary growth. It is antagonized by angiopoietin-2 which binds to the same endothelial cell-specific receptor Tie-2. TGF-β has among its many other effects a similar role as it is secreted by pericytes and stabilizes the basal membrane of newly built capillaries.

Pigment epithelium-derived factor is a cytokine that despite its name is produced in many human cells including endothelial cells and retinal pigment epithelial cells where it was originally detected. Among other effects it is a potent inhibitor of angiogenesis. It also has immunomodulatory features and contributes by this indirectly to prevention of neovascularization.

The vasoinhibins act as negative feedback regulators upon the effect of VEGF. They are upregulated in endothelial cells by VEGF and specifically inhibit migration and proliferation of these. Angiostatin also specifically inhibits proliferation of endothelial cells. It is a fragment of plasminogen and therefore exists as a plasma factor throughout the body.

Angiogenic Factors

The growth of new blood vessels is an important natural process occurring in the body, both in health and disease. Angiogenesis is a physiological process involving the growth of new blood vessels from preexisting vessels whereas vasculogenesis describes the formation of vascular structures from circulating or tissue-resident endothelial stem cells (angioblasts) which proliferate into de novo endothelial cells.

The healthy body controls angiogenesis through a series of 'on' and 'off' switches. The main 'on' switches are known as angiogenesis-stimulation growth factors, or simply angiogenic factors. Stimulation of angiogenesis is performed by various angiogenic proteins, including several growth factors, whereas the VEGF family has been demonstrated to be a major contributor to angiogenesis. Additionally, a large number of mediators exist which are involved in angiogenesis like insulin-like growth factor, the family of fibroblast growth factor, interleukins, angiopoietins, epidermal growth factor, transforming growth factors, platelet-derived growth factor, tumor necrosis factor-α and vascular endothelial cadherin.

The balance between angiogenesis and inhibitors of new vessel growth is controlled by a sophisticated interaction between different factors and mediators which will be described explicitly in the following chapter.

Prof. A.J. Augustin
Augenklinik
Moltkestrasse 90
DE–76133 Karlsruhe (Germany)
Tel. +49 721 9742001, Fax +49 721 9742009, E-Mail albertjaugustin@googlemail.com

Bandello F, Battaglia Parodi M (eds): Anti-VEGF.
Dev Ophthalmol. Basel, Karger, 2010, vol 46, pp 4–20

Mechanisms of Ocular Angiogenesis and Its Molecular Mediators

Martin J. Siemerink[a] · Albert J. Augustin[b] · Reinier O. Schlingemann[a,c]

[a]Ocular Angiogenesis Group, Department of Ophthalmology, Academic Medical Center, Amsterdam, The Netherlands; [b]Augenklinik, Karlsruhe, Germany, and [c]Netherlands Institute for Neuroscience, Royal Netherlands Academy of Arts and Sciences, Amsterdam, The Netherlands

Abstract

Angiogenesis is defined as the formation of new blood vessels from the existing vasculature. It is a highly coordinated process occurring during development of the retinal vasculature, ocular wound healing, and in pathological conditions. Complex interactions are involved between non-vascular and microvascular cells, such as endothelial cells and pericytes, via several angiogenic growth factors and inhibitors. Of these growth factors, vascular endothelial growth factor (VEGF) has emerged as the single most important causal agent of angiogenesis in health and disease in the eye. During the angiogenic process, endothelial cells shift from a homogeneous quiescent population into a population of heterogeneous phenotypes, each with a distinct cellular fate. So far, three angiogenic specialized phenotypes have been identified: (1) 'tip cells', which pick up guidance signals and migrate through the extracellular matrix; (2) 'stalk cells', which proliferate, form junctions, produce extracellular matrix, and form a lumen, and (3) 'phalanx cells', which do not proliferate, but align and form a smooth monolayer. Eventually, a robust mature new blood vessel is formed which is capable of supplying blood and oxygen to tissues. Pathological angiogenesis is a key component of several irreversible causes of blindness. In most of these conditions, angiogenesis is part of a wound healing response culminating, via an angiofibrotic switch, in fibrosis and scar formation which leads to blindness. Currently, VEGF-A antagonists are standard care in the treatment of exudative age-related macular degeneration, and have been found to be a valuable additional treatment strategy in several other vascular retinal diseases.

Blood vessels form an intricate hollow network of arteries, capillaries, and veins for the transport of liquids, solutes, gases, macromolecules, and cells throughout the vertebrate body. The vascular network is formed during early stages of development, and its correct and early function is absolutely critical for survival of the embryo. New blood vessels originate from endothelial precursor cells (angioblasts) by a process called vasculogenesis or from preexisting blood vessels by angiogenesis [1, 2]. Once a functional adult vascular system has been formed completely, blood vessels become quiescent. The growth potential of smaller blood vessels, however, is retained and is employed during wound healing and tissue regeneration.

Beyond its physiological roles, angiogenesis is also a hallmark of many pathological conditions, including neovascular diseases in the eye [3–5]. Excessive angiogenesis occurs when diseased cells produce abnormal amounts of angiogenic factors, overwhelming the effects of natural angiogenesis inhibitors. As the newly formed vessels mainly serve a role in a wound healing response, they usually do not restore the tissue integrity, but rather cause visual impairment when they are located in normally avascular, transparent tissues such as the cornea and vitreous. Strategies for inhibition of angiogenesis include approaches that can block the angiogenesis cascade at several steps [4, 6].

Angiogenesis: Mechanisms and Molecular Mediators

Endothelial Cell Differentiation

All blood vessels are lined by endothelial cells (ECs), which form the interface between circulating blood in the lumen and the rest of the vessel wall. Under normal conditions, ECs are a remarkably quiescent cell type, undergoing division approximately once every 1,000 days, but when activated, cell division can occur every 1–2 days [7]. Sprouting angiogenesis requires selection of ECs from an existing blood vessel which will be activated to form the new vessel, while at the same time, surrounding ECs remain quiescent in their current position. From recent studies a model has emerged in which ECs differentiate into three specialized cell types with distinct phenotypes during angiogenesis (fig. 1) [8–10]. First, a single 'tip cell' develops. This EC breaks down the basal lamina, emerges from its parent blood vessel and becomes the leading cell of the sprouting vessel. The tip cell migrates into the extracellular matrix and senses microenvironmental attractive and repulsive signals for guidance. Secondly, following directly behind the migrating tip cell, other ECs differentiate under the influence of the adjacent tip cell into 'stalk cells' that proliferate and bridge the gap between the tip cell and the parent vasculature. Stalk cells generate the blood vessel lumen through the formation of intracellular vacuoles, a process called 'lumenogenesis'. Thirdly, ECs behind the stalk cells differentiate into 'phalanx cells', and align in a smooth cobblestone monolayer, becoming the most inner cell layer in the new blood vessel. Phalanx cells no longer proliferate, express tight junctions and make contact with mural cells.

Angiogenesis Inducers and Inhibitors

Angiogenesis is tightly controlled by closely interacting angiogenic and angiostatic factors, and their balance ultimately determines if, where and when the 'angiogenic switch' is turned on with angiogenesis as the result [2, 9]. Over the past decades, numerous inducers of angiogenesis have been identified, including the members of

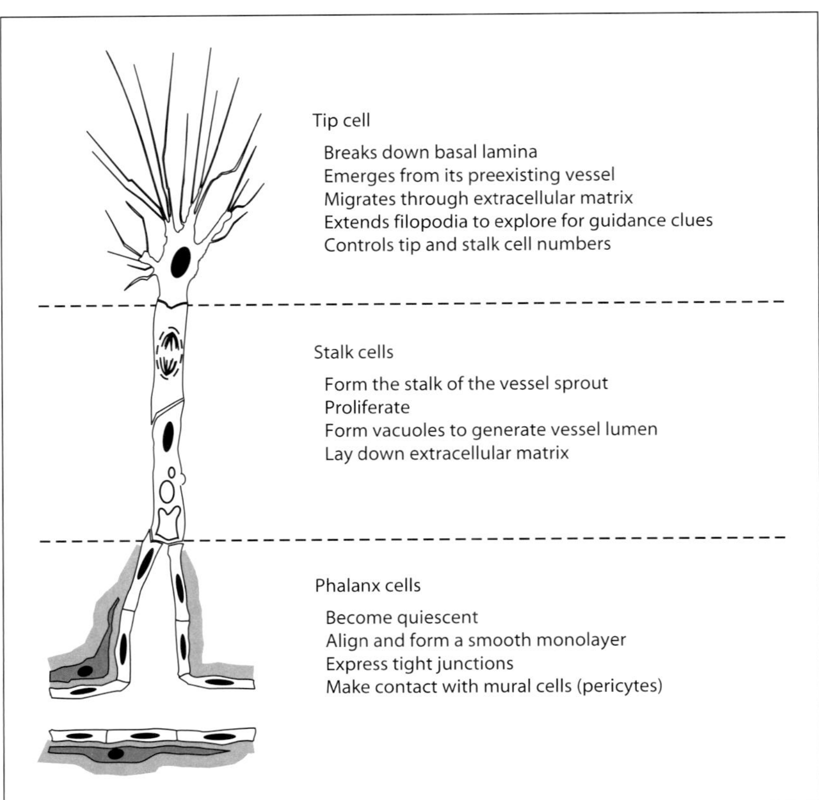

Fig. 1. Representative model of sprouting angiogenesis. At least three different angiogenic specialized endothelial cells (white) are required, each with a distinct cellular fate. In addition, the new blood vessel becomes surrounded by pericytes (dark gray) and a new basal lamina (light gray).

the vascular endothelial growth factor (VEGF) family, angiopoietins, transforming growth factors (TGF), epidermal growth factor (EGF), platelet-derived growth factor (PDGF), tumor necrosis factor-α (TNF-α), insulin-like growth factor (IGF), vascular endothelial-cadherin (VE-cadherin), interleukins and the members of the fibroblast growth factor (FGF) family. In addition, there is a plethora of growth factors, hormones and metabolites that have been reported to directly or indirectly stimulate physiological and pathological angiogenesis (table 1) [11, 12]. Not all of these factors are specific for ECs. Consistent with a major role for hypoxia in the overall process of angiogenesis, a large number of angiogenic factors involved in various stages of angiogenesis are independently responsive to hypoxia [13]. The VEGF family of proteins is the most important family of angiogenic factors that controls blood vessel formation.

Endogenous inhibitors of angiogenesis are defined as proteins or fragments of proteins that can inhibit the formation of blood vessels [14]. Angiogenesis inhibitors

Table 1. Major angiogenic factors

Protein (family)	Angiogenic members	Function(s)
Angiogenin		EC proliferation
Angiopoietins	Ang1	PC recruitment, vessel maturation
	Ang2	EC sprouting and migration, only in the presence of VEGF
Chemokine (C-C motif) ligands	CCL1 (I-309)	EC chemotaxis and differentiation
Chemokine (C-X-C motif) ligands	CXCL6, CXCL12	EC proliferation
Eph receptors and ephrins ligands	EphB4/ephrinB2	Arterial/venous differentiation, tip cell guidance
Epidermal growth factor	EGF	EC proliferation and migration
Erythropoietin	EPO	EC proliferation
Fibroblast growth factor family	aFGF, bFGF	EC proliferation and migration, ECM remodeling
Granulocyte-macrophage colony-stimulating factor	GM-CSF	EC proliferation and migration
Hepatocyte growth factor	HGF	EC proliferation and migration, PC proliferation
Hypoxia-inducible factor	HIF-1α, HIF-1β, HIF-2α	VEGF ↑
Insulin-like growth factor	IGF-1	EC proliferation, VEGF ↑
Integrins	Integrin αvβ3, Integrin αvβ5	Acquired for FGF induced angiogenesis, EC migration
Interleukins	IL-1, IL-6, IL-8, IL-13	EC proliferation, MMPs ↑
Matrix metalloproteinases	MMP-1, MMP-2, MMP-9	BL degradation, ECM remodeling
Monocyte chemotactic protein	MCP-1	Mediates TGF-β stimulated angiogenesis
Notch/delta-like ligand	Notch-1/Dll4	Tip/stalk cell regulation, arterial/venous differentiation
Plasminogen activator	PA1	EC migration
Platelet endothelial cell adhesion molecule	PECAM-1	EC tube formation and adhesion, tip cell filopodia formation
Platelet-activating factor	PAF	EC sprouting

Table 1. Continued

Protein (family)	Angiogenic members	Function(s)
Platelet-derived endothelial cell growth factor	PD-ECGF	EC proliferation
Platelet-derived growth factor	PDGF-BB	PC recruitment
Prostaglandins	PGE-1, PGE-2	EC proliferation
Stromal cell-derived factor	SDF-1	Angioblast migration
Thrombin		PDGF and PAF ↑, ECM remodeling
Transforming growth factor family	TGF-α, TGF-β	At low doses: EC proliferation and migration, ECM remodeling
Tumor necrosis factor	TNF-α	At low doses: EC proliferation and tube formation, tip cell 'priming'
Vascular endothelial cadherin	VE-cadherin	EC adhesion and proliferation
Vascular endothelial growth factor family	VEGF-A, VEGF-B, VEGF-C, VEGF-D, PlGF	Permeability ↑, EC sprouting, migration and proliferation, tip cell activation and guidance

EC = Endothelial cell, PC = pericyte, ECM = extracellular matrix, BL = basal lamina.

can be detected in circulating blood, suggesting that they function in the angiogenic switch as endogenous angiostatic regulators under physiological conditions. Various inhibitors of angiogenesis have been found in the body, including thrombospondin, angiostatin, endostatin and pigment epithelium-derived factor (PEDF) (table 2) [12, 14].

The VEGF Family and Their Receptors

In mammals, the VEGF family includes VEGF-A (also referred to in this review as VEGF), VEGF-B, placenta growth factor (PlGF), VEGF-C, VEGF-D, and the viral VEGF homologue VEGF-E. VEGFs bind selectively with different affinities to at least five distinct receptors: VEGF receptor-1 (VEGFR-1), also called Flt-1; VEGFR-2, also called Flk-1; VEGFR-3, also called Flt-4; neuropilin-1 (NRP-1), and NRP-2 [5, 15, 16]. The VEGFRs are members of the tyrosine-kinase receptor superfamily. Ligand binding to the extracellular immunoglobulin-like domain induces receptor dimerization. VEGFR-2 is considered to be the major receptor responsible for mediating the

Table 2. Major endogenous angiostatic factors

Protein (family)	Angiostatic members	Function(s)
Angiopoietins	Ang2	Antagonist of Ang1, vessel destabilization only in the *absence* of Ang1/VEGF
Angiostatin		EC proliferation ↓ and apoptosis ↑
Chemokine (C-C motif) ligand	CCL21	EC migration ↓
Chemokine (C-X-C motif) ligands	CXCL9, CXCL10, CXCL11, CXCL13	EC migration ↓, FGF ↓
	CXCL4	Inhibits VEGF and FGF binding
Endostatin		EC proliferation, migration and survival ↓, MMPs ↓
Interferons	IFN-α, IFN-β, IFN-γ	EC migration ↓, FGF ↓
Interleukins	IL-4, IL-10, IL-12, IL-18	EC migration ↓
Osteopontin		Integrins ↓
Pigment epithelium-derived factor	PEDF	EC migration and proliferation ↓
Plasminogen activator inhibitors	PAI-1, PAI-2	ECM remodeling ↓
Soluble neuropilin receptor	sNRP1	decoy receptor for VEGFs
Soluble vascular endothelial growth factor receptor	sVEGFR-1	decoy receptor for VEGFs
Thrombospondins	TSP1, TSP2	EC migration and proliferation ↓
Tissue inhibitor of metalloproteinases	TIMP-1, TIMP-2, TIMP-3, TIMP-4	EC migration ↓, ECM remodeling ↓
Transforming growth factor family	TGF-β	At high doses: EC proliferation and migration ↓, TIMPs ↑
Vascular endothelial growth inhibitor	VEGI	EC proliferation ↓
Vasculostatin		EC migration ↓
Vasostatin		EC proliferation ↓

EC = Endothelial cell, PC = pericyte, ECM = extracellular matrix, BL = basal lamina.

angiogenic effects of VEGF-A. The role of VEGFR-1 in angiogenesis remains controversial as its activation has been shown to both stimulate and suppress angiogenesis. However, soluble VEGFR-1 (sVEGFR-1) inhibits retinal angiogenesis in vivo [17]. VEGFR-3 is highly expressed in angiogenic sprouts in vivo and, like VEGFR-2, its signaling mediates angiogenesis [18]. NRPs are VEGF-A_{165}-, PlGF-, and VEGF-B-specific receptors, and form receptor complexes with VEGFRs: NRP-1 partners with VEGFR-2, whereas NRP-2 can form a complex with VEGFR-2 and VEGFR-3 [16].

VEGF-A, the best characterized and most studied of the VEGF family members, was originally described as a permeability factor, as it increases permeability of the endothelium through the formation of intercellular gaps and fenestrations. At least six human VEGF-A mRNA species, encoding VEGF-A isoforms of 121, 145, 165, 183, 189 and 206 amino acids, are produced by alternative splicing of the VEGF-A mRNA [15, 16]. In mouse, the VEGF-A isoforms are one amino acid shorter, i.e. VEGF-A_{120}, etc. It is widely accepted that VEGF-A is crucial for both vasculogenesis and angiogenesis: loss of only a single allele in mice or zebrafish is lethal, resulting in severe vascular defects and cardiovascular abnormalities [19]. VEGF-A exerts its biologic effect through interaction with VEGFR-1 and VEGFR-2, and the neuropilin receptors NRP-1 and NRP-2 [15].

VEGF-B yields two isoforms, VEGF-B_{167} and VEGF-B_{186} by alternative splicing, which signal through VEGFR-1 and NRP-1 [16]. VEGF-B is widely expressed in various tissues, including retina, but it is particularly abundant in the heart and skeletal muscle [15]. VEGF-B is able to directly stimulate EC growth and migration in vitro and in vivo [15]. However, the precise role of VEGF-B is not known, and genetic studies have revealed that VEGF-B-deficient mice are healthy and fertile, and do not display vascular defects, which indicate that VEGF-B is not involved or redundant in angiogenesis [15, 16].

PlGF is predominantly expressed in the placenta, heart and lungs, and binds VEGFR-1 and NRP-1 [16]. The binding of PlGF to VEGFR-1 leads to the formation of a complex between VEGFR-1 and -2, which enhances VEGF-A signaling and stimulates angiogenesis [15]. PlGF upregulates the expression of VEGF-A, FGF-2, PDGF-B, matrix metalloproteinases (MMPs) and other angiogenic factors, suggesting that ECs are able to enhance their own responsiveness to VEGF-A by producing PlGF. Furthermore, PlGF can promote blood vessel maturation via the recruitment of mural cells [15].

VEGF-C and VEGF-D both bind VEGFR-2, but with a lower affinity than they bind to VEGFR-3. Like VEGF-A, both VEGF-C and VEGF-D are able to stimulate the migration and proliferation of ECs in vitro and in vivo [15]. VEGFR-3 expression is more abundant on tip cells than on stalk cells [18], whereas VEGFR-3 expression is absent on phalanx cells. It has been suggested that VEGF-C may cooperate with VEGF-A to activate ECs for angiogenic sprouting via VEGFR-2/VEGFR-3 receptor complex.

The viral VEGF homologue VEGF-E is a potent angiogenic factor as well [16].

Matrix Degradation

Before ECs can grow out from preexisting vessels, the EC basal lamina must be degraded and the extracellular matrix needs to be remodeled [8, 9, 12]. This is achieved by a complex interplay of angiogenic growth factors, mural cells, and ECs. Acidic and basic FGFs (aFGF and bFGF, respectively) and VEGF stimulate the production of collagenase and MMPs, and upregulate urokinase-type plasminogen activator in ECs [20]. Collagenases are enzymes that break the peptide bonds in collagens; urokinase-type plasminogen activator converts plasminogen into plasmin, leading to fibrinolysis; and MMPs are capable of degrading all kinds of extracellular matrix proteins. Furthermore, low-dose stimulation by TGF-β upregulates proteases in ECs [21]. At the same time, FGFs and VEGF downregulate endogenous inhibitors of proteolytic enzymes such as tissue inhibitors of metalloproteinases (TIMPs) [20].

Tip and Stalk Cell Regulation

The selection of an endothelial tip cell from a population of quiescent ECs has to be tightly regulated since excessive tip cell formation would result in a poorly patterned, hyperdense vessel network that may not be functional. Clearly both tip and stalk cells are stimulated by the same growth factor, VEGF, and both respond through VEGFR-2 signaling [9, 10, 22]. However, their behavior is very different and in vivo studies show that tip and stalk cells carry a differential transcriptional signature [9, 10, 22]. In tip cells, VEGFR-2 signaling induces the expression of the Notch ligand delta-like 4 (DLL4), which is transported to the cell membrane and binds to Notch receptors on adjacent ECs [22–26]. After ligand binding, Notch is cleaved in these future stalk cells, generating the Notch intracellular domain that acts as a transcriptional regulator. In these stalk cells, notch activation downregulates the expression of VEGFR-2, VEGFR-3 and NRP-1, while inducing the transcription of VEGFR-1 and its soluble splice variant sVEGFR-1 [24–26]. Experimental inhibition of Dll4-Notch1 signaling raised the number of tip cells during early postembryonic angiogenesis, leading to increased sprout densities and change in vascular patterning [22]. Overactivation of Notch signaling, on the other hand, reduced the migratory behavior of ECs [22]. Other Notch ligands expressed by sprouting vessels are Jagged1 and Dll1, and loss of each of these also results in vascular defects. However, Dll4 is the only ligand expressed in tip cells, whereas Jagged1 and Dll1 are present in stalk cells [27]. These data indicate that the graded distribution of VEGF together with Dll-Notch signaling regulates angiogenic behavior of ECs by limiting the number of cells that become tip cell.

Endothelial Proliferation

The stimulatory effects of VEGFs on EC proliferation have been well reported in vitro and in vivo [5, 16]. Interestingly, during angiogenesis, adjacent ECs exhibit distinct cellular behavior patterns, even when exposed to a similar degree of VEGF-A, indicating that several other key molecules are involved in EC differentiation into tip cells, stalk cells or phalanx cells [22]. Co-expression of NRPs with VEGFR-2 is typical for endothelial tip cells, where it enhances VEGF-A binding to VEGFR-2, VEGFR-2 phosphorylation and VEGF-induced signaling, all of which are required for migration. In stalk cells, where NRP expression is absent, VEGF-A signaling via VEGFR-2 promotes proliferation but not migration [8, 10, 22].

At low doses, TGF-β contributes to the angiogenic switch by upregulating angiogenic factors in ECs, but it has inhibitory effects at higher concentrations [21]. TGF-β family ligands stimulate type II receptors that phosphorylate type I receptors (such as activin receptor-like kinase (ALK)) and activate the downstream signaling Smads. Endoglin is a type III receptor, which facilitates ALK1/TGF-β signaling in ECs, and ALK1/Endoglin/TGF-β signaling also promotes EC proliferation and migration. Addition of a neutralizing antibody against TGF-β strongly inhibited angiogenesis in vitro and in vivo [21]. The angiogenic effects of TNF-α are similar to those of TGF-β, as it promotes EC proliferation and tube formation in lower doses, but inhibits angiogenesis in higher doses [28].

Angiopoietin-2 (Ang-2) can act as an angiogenic factor depending on the presence of co-stimulatory molecules. For example, in the presence of VEGF, Ang-2 induces migration and proliferation of ECs by binding to the Tie2 receptor and thereby blocking Tie2 signaling of angiopoietin-1 (Ang-1). In the absence of VEGF, however, Ang-2 causes apoptosis of ECs and regression of blood vessels. Ang-1 has an antagonizing effect on Tie2 and inhibits EC proliferation. Ang-1 secreted by pericytes binds to Tie2 on ECs, and is important for maintenance of vessel integrity and quiescence.

Several other molecules have been reported to stimulate EC proliferation, including FGFs, EGF, CXC chemokines and insulin-like growth factor-1 (IGF-1) [12, 29].

Endothelial Cell-Cell Interaction

EC junctions are composed of a complex network of adhesion proteins that are linked to the intracellular cytoskeletal network and signaling molecules. VE-cadherin is specifically localized to the inter-EC junction, and is known to be required for maintaining a restrictive endothelial barrier. VE-cadherin is critical for proper vascular development: VE-cadherin-null mice die in early embryonic stages because of vascular defects [30]. The functions of cadherins are modulated by catenins, which bind with the intracellular tail of the cadherins. After activation of VEGFR-2 by VEGF, catenins become highly phosphorylated, leading to loss of cell-cell junctions, allowing EC to differentiate and move from their current position. Later on during angiogenesis, the phosphorylation of catenins decreases, allowing restabilization of EC cell-cell junctions and the differentiation into quiescent phalanx cells.

Platelet EC adhesion molecule-1 (PECAM-1) is expressed on ECs, and like VE-cadherin, it is enriched in intercellular junctions. PECAM-1 mediated cell-cell junctions are necessary for the organization of ECs in to tubular networks in vitro, and PECAM-1 has been shown to stimulate the formation of tip cell filopodia in vivo [31].

Blood Vessel Guidance

Endothelial tip cells pick up attractive or repulsive signals from the tissue environment and translate them into a dynamic process of adhesion and de-adhesion, leading to migration. In this process the tip cell forms lamellipodia (short cytoskeletal projection) and filopodia (long finger-like plasma membrane extensions) [8]. Lamellipodia are located on the mobile edge of the cell. They adhere and connect the intracellular cytoskeleton to the extracellular matrix, allowing stress fibers of actin/myosin filaments to pull the cell forward. Filopodia protrude from the lamellipodial actin network and function as antennae with which tip cells probe their environment. The main regulators of filopodia and lamellipodia formation are members of the Rho small GTPases, which are induced by VEGF [32].

An extracellular VEGF-A gradient appears to be a strong attractant for migrating ECs via binding to VEGFR-2 and NRPs, which are prominent on tip cell filopodia. An important biological property of the different VEGF-A isoforms is their heparin and heparan-sulfate-binding ability. The larger VEGF-A isoforms bind very tightly to heparin and remain sequestered in the extracellular matrix, whereas the shorter VEGF-A isoforms are freely diffusible. It is well established that VEGF-A_{189} and VEGF-A_{165} function as a chemoattractive signal that promote the polarized extension of tip cell filopodia, whereas VEGF-A_{121} can support EC proliferation but not tip cell guidance [22, 33].

Furthermore, the function of endothelial tip cells bears remarkable similarity to that of axonal growth cones. Blood vessels and nerve fibers course throughout the body alongside one another and it has been reported that during embryogenesis, their patterning is guided in large part by similar attractive and repulsive guidance cues. Thus far, four major families of receptors have been shown to regulate guidance events during axonal and vascular morphogenesis: Plexin/NRP complexes with their ligands class 3 semaphorins; 'uncoordinated-5' (UNC5) family and 'deleted in colorectal cancer' (DCC) with their ligands netrins; 'Roundabout' (Robo) with their ligands Slits, and Eph and their ligands ephrins [9, 33, 34].

Lumen Formation

While migrating, the leading tip cell creates a tunnel throughout the extracellular matrix space. Behind the tip cell, stalk cells flatten onto the wall of this tube-like space in the extracellular matrix, resulting in an apical and basal face of the endothelium. Stalk cells form large intracellular vacuoles by fusion of intracellular vesicles, mediated by integrins, which fuse together to form a lumen [9, 35]. Multiple integrins as well as the transcription factor myocyte enhancer binding factor 2C (MEF2C) are able to participate in vesicle formation and fusion in vitro [35]. EC interactions with the extracellular matrix establish signaling cascades downstream of integrin ligation leading to activation of the Rho family of GTPases. Inhibition of Rho GTPases results in complete blockade of EC vacuole and lumen formation in vitro [35].

Recruitment of Mural Cells and Maturation

After the initial vessel formation through angiogenesis, determination of artery or vein identity is regulated by a variety of molecular factors which specify EC fate. Distinct arterial and venous molecular markers are evident even before the initiation of circulatory flow, suggesting that molecular determinants play a critical role in arterial/venous differentiation. Several relevant genes have now been identified in vivo, including the Hedgehog family of secreted morphogens, notch signaling, NRPs, EphB4, ephrinB2, and VEGF [36].

The two major classes of mural cells are the vascular smooth muscle cells, which coat veins and arteries, and the pericytes, which are present in variable amounts around capillaries. The mural cells are indispensable to provide survival and antiproliferative factors that stabilize the newly-formed vessel. However, the hypothesis that pericyte loss initializes the first steps of angiogenesis whereas pericyte recruitment only occurs at the completion of angiogenesis is controversial, since many pericytes are found to be present in endothelial sprouts in vivo [37].

The development and the recruitment of vascular mural cells require the function of PDGF signaling, Ang-1 and its receptor Tie-2, and Ephrin-Eph interaction. PDGFs exist as heterodimers (PDGF-AB) or homodimers composed of chains A and B. Endothelial tip cells from growing vascular sprouts generate a PDGF-B concentration gradient that promotes the recruitment of pericytes expressing the PDGF-B receptor [37, 38]. This in turn activates TGF-β in pericytes, which introduces the production of basal lamina components that are required for final blood vessel maturation and stabilization [21].

Ang-1, expressed by perivascular cells, binds to and activates the Tie2 receptor, thereby stimulating mural cell attachment. In agreement, a poor association between ECs and surrounding mural cells was seen in Ang-1 and Tie2 knockouts. Ang-2 was shown to have an antagonizing effect on Tie2 inducing pericyte loss and capillary degeneration in the retina. However, endothelial expression of Tie2 has been observed on newly formed vessels that are still immature [37].

Retinal Circulation

Retinal Vascular System

The retina has a dual vascular supply: the outer one-third of the retina is supplied from the choroidal circulation and the inner two-thirds by the central retinal artery. The choroidal arteries pierce the sclera around the optic nerve and fan out to form the choriocapillaris, providing nutrients and oxygen to the retinal pigment epithelium and the photoreceptors in the outer part of retina. The corresponding venous lobules drain into the venules and veins that run anterior towards the equator of the eyeball to enter the vortex veins. The vortex veins penetrate the sclera and ultimately merge into the ophthalmic vein. The central retinal artery pierces the optic nerve close to the eyeball, emerges at the optic disk, and sends 4 main branches over the human retina, lying close to the inner limiting membrane. Each of the 4 branches of the central retinal artery supplies one quadrant of the inner retina. The venous equivalent of the central retinal artery is the retinal vein. The anatomy of the veins of the orbit of the eye varies between individuals. In some the central retinal vein drains into the superior ophthalmic vein whereas in others it drains directly into the cavernous sinus [39,40].

Unique Characteristics of Retinal Circulation

Regulation of the microenvironment of the retina, e.g. the controlled fluid and molecular movement between the ocular vascular bed and the retinal tissues, is fundamental for appropriate retinal function and vision. Therefore, the retina has a unique blood-retinal barrier that separates the retina from the circulating blood [41]. The blood-retinal barrier is formed by complex tight junctions of retinal capillary ECs (the inner barrier) and retinal pigment epithelial cells (the outer barrier), corresponding to the two main circulations. The choroidal capillaries themselves are fenestrated, like most of the highly permeable capillaries throughout the human body. Retinal capillary ECs express a variety of unique transporters which play a key role in the influx transport of essential molecules and the efflux transport of neurotransmitter metabolites, toxins, and drugs [41]. Therefore, systemic drug administration is not suitable for the treatment of retinal diseases because of poor drug permeability across the blood-retinal barrier.

Retinal circulation is characterized by a low blood flow and a high level of oxygen extraction; arteriovenous difference in pO_2 is about 40% [42]. Autonomic nerve endings extend to the uvea and the extraocular part of the retinal blood vessels, but not to the intraocular segments of the retinal blood vessels. Therefore, retinal arterial tone is largely regulated by local factors such as local variations in perfusion pressure and in pO_2, pCO_2 and pH [42]. The presence of mechanisms that autoregulate retinal circulation may well reflect important survival strategies for the retina which are not yet fully understood.

Development of the Retinal Vasculature

During embryogenesis, the vascular network that supplies the retina undergoes dramatic changes and reorganization [39]. The choroidal vasculature develops in an early stage and is preceded by a peak of VEGF-A production by the retinal pigment epithelium, suggesting that VEGF-A is involved in the development of the choroidal vasculature [43]. Initially, the inner part of the eye is metabolically supported by the hyaloidal vasculature, an arterial network in the vitreous. Blood enters through the central hyaloid artery in the optic nerve, runs through hyaloid vessels in the vitreous and then exits through an annular collection vessel at the front of the eye. The hyaloid vessel system is a dense, but transient intraocular circulatory system that undergoes progressive and nearly complete regression during the latest stage of ocular development as the lens, the vitreous and the retina mature. Due to the natural regression of the hyaloidal vasculature, as well as increasing metabolic demands of maturing neurons, the retina becomes hypoxic, and therefore the formation of the retinal vasculature is induced.

Retinal Angioblasts

Recent observations have suggested that the initial human retinal vasculature develops by differentiation, and organization of vascular precursor cells that are CD39+ (angioblast marker) and CD34–/CD31– (EC markers) at around 14 weeks of gestation [44]. These cells seem to emerge from a pool of precursor cells that are CXCR4+/c-Kit+ (angioblast receptors), and were found in the neuroblastic layer of human embryonic retina at 7 weeks of gestation. CD39+/CXCR4+/c-Kit+ cells start to migrate anteriorly into the retinal nerve fiber layer where stroma-derived factor-1 (SDF-1, the ligand for CXCR4) and stem cell factor (SCF, the ligand for c-Kit) levels are at their highest. With apparent migration of these vascular precursors, the expression of c-Kit declines and differentiation into angioblasts and alignment with nerve fibers occurs. A gradient of SDF-1 towards the ora serrata suggests that the angioblasts migrate towards the higher concentration. CXCR4 expression is regulated by SCF, FGF-2 and VEGF, and angioblasts continue to express CXCR4 until they become ECs that are CD34+/CD31+. These results suggest, at least in part, that vasculogenesis might contribute to growth of the primordial vessels in the central retina [44, 45]. However, the identification and lineage of angioblasts within the developing retina is still controversial [46].

Retinal Angiogenesis

After formation of primordial vessels, new blood vessels sprout into the retina by means of angiogenesis, forming the vasculature of the inner retina. Retinal angiogenesis begins in the most superficial retinal layer at the optic nerve head, and radiates outwards from this central point [3, 39, 45]. The superficial plexus develops in a centrifugal fashion across the inner surface of the retina, with the exception of the primate fovea from which blood vessels are excluded. Retinal angiogenesis is closely regulated by supply and demand of oxygen. High oxygen tension suppresses hypoxia-induced VEGF production, and less VEGF results in less blood vessel growth [3, 39]. Additional capillary networks in deeper retinal layers then arise by sprouting from the superficial arteries to form the deeper vascular plexus. Vascular pruning in the developing retina results from EC migration from retracting vessels into the surrounding newly developing vessels. The process of natural pruning can be accelerated by experimental exposure to hyperoxia [3]. The process of retinal vascular development is completed shortly before birth in humans, and a few weeks after birth in several other mammalian species including rodents. With development of the capillary plexuses and the resulting increase in oxygen tension, a capillary-free zone develops around the major blood vessels, followed by vessel retraction in the superficial plexus [40].

Vascular Patterning

The process of sprouting angiogenesis during development of the retinal vasculature is preceded by an invasion of migrating astrocytes in a centrifugal fashion across the inner surface of the retina [3, 22, 40, 46, 47]. Ganglion cells secrete PDGF-A to stimulate proliferation of astrocytes [48, 49]. The retinal vascular plexus initially forms superimposed on the astrocyte network. Astrocytes at the leading edge and immediately ahead of the vascular plexus secrete high levels of VEGF-A compared to more distally located astrocytes that already have established contact with ECs. During this burst of angiogenesis, all endothelial tip cells are closely attached to astrocytes and their filopodia orientate along the astrocyte cell bodies and processes. Experimental overexpression of PDGF-A in ganglion cells resulted in a large increase in the number of retinal astrocytes and subsequent overgrowth of the retinal vasculature in vivo [49]. However, blocking PDGF-A receptor reduced astrocyte network formation but showed only small changes in blood vessel formation [49].

Pathological Ocular Angiogenesis

What Is Unique in Ocular Angiogenesis?

Several ocular diseases are hallmarked by angiogenesis, including diabetic retinopathy, age-related macular degeneration, and retinopathy of prematurity [3, 5, 46, 50]. In all these conditions, angiogenesis is probably stimulated by local tissue hypoxia resulting from neuronal metabolism, with varying contributions from inflammatory signals and oxidative stress. In retinal neovascularization, VEGF plays a central role [3, 5, 51]. At least five retinal cell types have the capacity to produce and secrete VEGF. These include the retinal pigmented epithelium, astrocytes, Müller cells, ECs and ganglion cells. However, they differ widely in their responses to hypoxia; in vitro studies show that Müller cells and astrocytes generally produce the greatest amounts of VEGF under hypoxic conditions [1, 22, 43]. The two most important forms of ocular angiogenesis are preretinal angiogenesis, originating from the retinal vasculature, and subretinal (or choroidal) neovascularization.

Preretinal Angiogenesis

Preretinal angiogenesis occurs as a final common pathway in several diseases associated with capillary non-perfusion and local retinal ischemia, including diabetic retinopathy. Angiogenesis is induced by the ischemic retinal areas, and ultimately results in the formation of large contractile fibrovascular membranes within the vitreous cavity. These membranes and the associated hemorrhages cause blindness by obscuration of the visual axis and retinal detachment. When the retinal ischemia is widespread, angiogenesis and scarring can also occur on the iris and cause an untreatable form of glaucoma. Destruction of the ischemic retinal areas with laser can be effective in inducing regression and fibrosis of the newly formed vessels.

Subretinal Angiogenesis

Subretinal, or choroidal neovascularization, results from a series of pathological events affecting the retinal pigment epithelium, Bruch's membrane, and the choroid. Typically, subretinal angiogenesis is a wound healing response that occurs only when an anatomical discontinuation of Bruch's membrane is present, in combination with a driving force such as inflammation, hypoxia, and oxidative stress. For most conditions it is unknown to what extent these three mechanisms contribute to the initiation of subretinal angiogenesis. Subretinal angiogenesis is a hallmark of age-related macular degeneration, occurring either between the retinal pigment epithelium and Bruch's membrane (occult choroidal neovascularization), or between the retinal pigment epithelium and the neuroretina (classic choroidal neovascularization).

New vessels formed by subretinal angiogenesis can later regress, leaving an atrophic retinal area, or the wound healing can progress with formation of a fibrotic scar. In both cases, the overlying neuroretina will slowly degenerate, leading to loss of sharp sight, contrast sensitivity, and color vision.

Ocular Angiogenesis and Wound Healing Responses

In most instances, pathological ocular angiogenesis is a wound healing-like response in which the formation of blood vessels is accompanied by influx of inflammatory cells, followed by myofibroblast formation [52]. Therefore, during disease progression, the angiogenic phase can be followed by a fibrotic phase. It has been shown that VEGF-driven angiogenesis upregulates profibrotic factors such as TGF-β_1 and connective tissue growth factor (CTGF) [53]. CTGF levels strongly correlate with degree of fibrosis in vitreoretinal conditions [52]. When the balance between the angiogenic (VEGF) and fibrotic (CTGF) factors shifts to a certain threshold ratio in favor of fibrosis, the 'angiofibrotic switch' occurs and fibrosis and scarring develop [52]. Administration of anti-VEGF drugs to patients as a therapy to regress neovascularization could therefore lead to a temporary increase in fibrosis, a phenomenon that is indeed observed in the clinic.

References

1 Patan S: Vasculogenesis and angiogenesis as mechanisms of vascular network formation, growth and remodeling. J Neurooncol 2000;50:1–15.

2 Risau W: Mechanisms of angiogenesis. Nature 1997; 386:671–674.

3 Gariano RF, Gardner TW: Retinal angiogenesis in development and disease. Nature 2005;438:960–966.

4 Schlingemann RO, Witmer AN: Treatment of retinal diseases with VEGF antagonists. Prog Brain Res 2009;175:253–267.

5 Witmer AN, Vrensen GFJM, van Noorden CJF, Schlingemann RO: Vascular endothelial growth factors and angiogenesis in eye disease. Prog Retin Eye Res 2003;22:1–29.

6 Andreoli CM, Miller JW: Antivascular endothelial growth factor therapy for ocular neovascular disease. Curr Opin Ophthalmol 2007;18:502–508.

7 Cines DB, Pollak ES, Buck CA, Loscalzo J, Zimmerman GA, McEver RP, et al: Endothelial cells in physiology and in the pathophysiology of vascular disorders. Blood 1998;91:3527–3561.

8 De Smet F, Segura I, De Bock K, Hohensinner PJ, Carmeliet P: Mechanisms of vessel branching filopodia on endothelial tip cells lead the way. Arterioscler Thromb Vasc Biol 2009;29:639–649.
9 Adams RH, Alitalo K: Molecular regulation of angiogenesis and lymphangiogenesis. Nat Rev Mol Cell Biol 2007;8:464–478.
10 Le Noble F, Klein C, Tintu A, Pries A, Buschmann I: Neural guidance molecules, tip cells, and mechanical factors in vascular development. Cardiovasc Res 2008;78:232–241.
11 Otrock ZK, Mahfouz RAR, Makarm JA, Shamseddine AI: Understanding the biology of angiogenesis: review of the most important molecular mechanisms. Blood Cells Mol Dis 2007;39:212–220.
12 Distler JHW, Hirth A, Kurowska-Stolarska M, Gay RE, Gay S, Distler O: Angiogenic and angiostatic factors in the molecular control of angiogenesis. Q J Nucl Med 2003;47:149–161.
13 Fong GH: Regulation of angiogenesis by oxygen sensing mechanisms. J Mol Med 2009;87:549–560.
14 Tabruyn SP, Griffioen AW: Molecular pathways of angiogenesis inhibition. Biochem Biophys Res Commun 2007;355:1–5.
15 Tammela T, Enholm B, Alitalo K, Paavonen K: The biology of vascular endothelial growth factors. Cardiovasc Res 2005;65:550–563.
16 Holmes DIR, Zachary I: The vascular endothelial growth factor family: angiogenic factors in health and disease. Genome Biol 2005;6.
17 Aiello LP, Pierce EA, Foley ED, Takagi H, Chen H, Riddle L, et al: Suppression of retinal neovascularization in vivo by inhibition of vascular endothelial growth-factor (VEGF) using soluble VEGF-receptor chimeric proteins. Proc Natl Acad Sci USA 1995;92: 10457–10461.
18 Witmer AN, van Blijswijk BC, Dai J, Hofman P, Partanen TA, Vrensen GFJM, et al: VEGFR-3 in adult angiogenesis. J Pathol 2001;195:490–497.
19 Carmeliet P, Ferreira V, Breier G, Pollefeyt S, Kieckens L, Gertsenstein M, et al: Abnormal blood vessel development and lethality in embryos lacking a single VEGF allele. Nature 1996;380:435–439.
20 Presta M, Dell'Era P, Mitola S, Moroni E, Ronca R, Rusnati M: Fibroblast growth factor/fibroblast growth factor receptor system in angiogenesis. Cytokine Growth Factor Rev 2005;16:159–178.
21 Goumans MJ, Liu Z, ten Dijke P: TGF-β signaling in vascular biology and dysfunction. Cell Res 2009;19: 116–127.
22 Gerhardt H, Golding M, Fruttiger M, Ruhrberg C, Lundkvist A, Abramsson A, et al: VEGF guides angiogenic sprouting utilizing endothelial tip cell filopodia. J Cell Biol 2003;161:1163–1177.
23 Hellstrom M, Phng LK, Hofmann JJ, Wallgard E, Coultas L, Lindblom P, et al: Dll4 signalling through Notch1 regulates formation of tip cells during angiogenesis. Nature 2007;445:776–780.
24 Leslie JD, Ariza-McNaughton L, Bermange AL, McAdow R, Johnson SL, Lewis J: Endothelial signalling by the Notch ligand delta-like 4 restricts angiogenesis. Development 2007;134:839–844.
25 Harrington LS, Sainson RCA, Williams CK, Taylor JM, Shi W, Li JL, et al: Regulation of multiple angiogenic pathways by D114 and Notch in human umbilical vein endothelial cells. Microvasc Res 2008;75:144–154.
26 Hainaud P, Contreres JO, Villemain A, Liu LX, Plouet J, Tobelem G, et al: The role of the vascular endothelial growth factor-delta-like 4 ligand/ Notch4-ephrin B2 cascade in tumor vessel remodeling and endothelial cell functions. Cancer Res 2006; 66:8501–8510.
27 Roca C, Adams RH: Regulation of vascular morphogenesis by Notch signaling. Genes Dev 2007;21: 2511–2524.
28 Sainson RCA, Johnston DA, Chu HC, Holderfield MT, Nakatsu MN, Crampton SP, et al: TNF primes endothelial cells for angiogenic sprouting by inducing a tip cell phenotype. Blood 2008;111:4997–5007.
29 Otrock ZK, Mahfouz RAR, Makarm JA, Shamseddine AI: Understanding the biology of angiogenesis: review of the most important molecular mechanisms. Blood Cells Mol Dis 2007;39:212–220.
30 Wallez Y, Vilgrain I, Huber P: Angiogenesis: the VE-cadherin switch. Trends Cardiovasc Med 2006; 16:55–59.
31 Cao GY, Fehrenbach ML, Williams JT, Finklestein JM, Zhu JX, DeLisser HM: Angiogenesis in platelet endothelial cell adhesion molecule-1-null mice. Am J Pathol 2009;175:903–915.
32 Mattila PK, Lappalainen P: Filopodia: molecular architecture and cellular functions. Nat Rev Mol Cell Biol 2008;9:446–454.
33 Carmeliet P: Blood vessels and nerves: common signals, pathways and diseases. Nat Rev Genet 2003;4: 710–720.
34 Larrivee B, Freitas C, Suchting S, Brunet I, Eichmann A: Guidance of vascular development lessons from the nervous system. Circ Res 2009;104:428–441.
35 Iruela-Arispe ML, Davis GE: Cellular and molecular mechanisms of vascular lumen formation. Dev Cell 2009;16:222–231.
36 Swift MR, Weinstein BM: Arterial-venous specification during development. Circ Res 2009;104:576–588.

37 Witmer AN, van Blijswijk BC, van Noorden CJF, Vrensen GFJM, Schlingemann RO: In vivo angiogenic phenotype of endothelial cells and pericytes induced by vascular endothelial growth factor-A. J Histochem Cytochem 2004;52:39–52.
38 Penfold PL, Provis JM, Madigan MC, Vandriel D, Billson FA: Angiogenesis in normal human retinal development – the involvement of astrocytes and macrophages. Graefes Arch Clin Exp Ophthalmol 1990;228:255–263.
39 Saint-Geniez M, D'Amore PA: Development and pathology of the hyaloid, choroidal and retinal vasculature. Int J Dev Biol 2004;48:1045–1058.
40 Provis JM: Development of the primate retinal vasculature. Prog Retin Eye Res 2001;20:799–821.
41 Kaur C, Foulds WS, Ling EA: Blood-retinal barrier in hypoxic ischaemic conditions: basic concepts, clinical features and management. Prog Retin Eye Res 2008;27:622–647.
42 Hardy P, Beauchamp M, Sennlaub F, Gobeil F, Tremblay L, Mwaikambo B, et al: New insights into the retinal circulation: inflammatory lipid mediators in ischemic retinopathy. Prostaglandins Leukot Essent Fatty Acids 2005;72:301–325.
43 Gogat K, Le Gat L, Van den Berghe L, Marchant D, Kobetz A, Gadin S, et al: VEGF and KDR gene expression during human embryonic and fetal eye development. Invest Ophthalmol Vis Sci 2004;45:7–14.
44 Hasegawa T, McLeod DS, Prow T, Merges C, Grebe R, Lutty GA: Vascular precursors in developing human retina. Invest Ophthalmol Vis Sci 2008;49:2178–2192.
45 Hughes S, Yang HJ, Chan-Ling T: Vascularization of the human fetal retina: roles of vasculogenesis and angiogenesis. Invest Ophthalmol Vis Sci 2000;41:1217–1228.
46 Gariano RF: Cellular mechanisms in retinal vascular development. Prog Retin Eye Res 2003;22:295–306.
47 Chan-Ling T, McLeod DS, Hughes S, Baxter L, Chu Y, Hasegawa T, et al: Astrocyte-endothelial cell relationships during human retinal vascular development. Invest Ophthalmol Vis Sci 2004;45:2020–2032.
48 Sandercoe TM, Madigan MC, Billson FA, Penfold PL, Provis JM: Astrocyte proliferation during development of the human retinal vasculature. Exp Eye Res 1999;69:511–523.
49 Fruttiger M, Calver AR, Kruger WH, Mudhar HS, Michalovich D, Takakura N, et al: PDGF mediates a neuron-astrocyte interaction in the developing retina. Neuron 1996;17:1117–1131.
50 Campochiaro PA, Hackett SF: Ocular neovascularization: a valuable model system. Oncogene 2003;22:6537–6548.
51 Blaauwgeers HGT, Hotkamp BW, Rutten H, Witmer AN, Koolwijk P, Partanen TA, et al: Polarized vascular endothelial growth factor secretion by human retinal pigment epithelium and localization of vascular endothelial growth factor receptors on the inner choriocapillaris – evidence for a trophic paracrine relation. Am J Pathol 1999;155:421–428.
52 Kuiper EJ, Van Nieuwenhoven FA, de Smet MD, van Meurs JC, Tanck MW, Oliver N, et al: The angiofibrotic switch of VEGF and CTGF in proliferative diabetic retinopathy. PLoS One 2008;3:e2675.
53 Kuiper EJ, Hughes JM, Van Geest RJ, Vogels IMC, Goldschmeding R, van Noorden CJF, et al: Effect of VEGF-A on expression of profibrotic growth factor and extracellular matrix genes in the retina. Invest Ophthalmol Vis Sci 2007;48:4267–4276.

Prof. Dr. R.O. Schlingemann
Medical Retina Unit and Ocular Angiogenesis Group, Department of Ophthalmology
Academic Medical Center, University of Amsterdam, A2-122
PO Box 22660, NL–1100 DD Amsterdam (The Netherlands)
Tel. +31 205 663 682, Fax +31 205 669 048, E-Mail r.schlingemann@amc.uva.nl

Bandello F, Battaglia Parodi M (eds): Anti-VEGF.
Dev Ophthalmol. Basel, Karger, 2010, vol 46, pp 21–38

Antivascular Endothelial Growth Factors in Age-Related Macular Degeneration

Ursula Schmidt-Erfurth · Andreas Pollreisz · Christoph Mitsch · Matthias Bolz

Department of Ophthalmology and Optometry, Medical University Vienna, Vienna, Austria

Abstract

Age-related macular degeneration (AMD) is the leading cause of irreversible vision loss in adults aged over 50 years in developed countries. Until recently, argon laser photocoagulation and photodynamic therapy (PDT) were the only treatments available for the neovascular form of AMD. The introduction of new intravitreally injectable inhibitors of vascular endothelial growth factor (VEGF) revolutionized the management of the wet form. Pegaptanib was the first anti-VEGF agent to be approved by the US Food and Drug Administration (FDA) for use in neovascular AMD. The VISION study showed that patients receiving pegaptanib lost vision in a smaller rate than those treated with conventional care. Bevacizumab is a full-length recombinant humanized monoclonal antibody which binds to all isoforms of VEGF-A. It is licensed for the intravenous administration for the treatment of malignant solid tumors and is available for off-label use in the treatment of AMD-related CNV. Numerous retrospective studies have shown beneficial effects of bevacizumab in patients with neovascular AMD. Ranibizumab is a recombinant, humanized antibody antigen-binding fragment (F_{ab}) that binds to all known active forms of VEGF-A. The US FDA approved ranibizumab for treatment of all subtypes of choroidal neovascularization secondary to AMD. VEGF trap is a pharmacologically engineered protein that binds VEGF with higher affinity than pegaptanib or ranibizumab and thus prevents VEGF binding to its cellular receptor offering a theoretically longer interval between necessary treatments. A number of studies have shown that OCT imaging allows identification of functionally relevant factors like subretinal fluid or retinal thickness, which are important for the establishment of optimized individual dosing regimen during anti-angiogenesis therapies.

Age-related macular degeneration (AMD) is the leading cause of irreversible vision loss in adults aged over 50 years in developed countries. Large population studies report prevalence rates of early AMD between 5.8 and 15.1% [1, 2]. Giving demographic development in the aging of the population, its prevalence will increase dramatically in the following years [3, 4]. AMD should therefore not only be regarded as a medical problem but also as a major socioeconomic burden.

AMD is a term used to summarize different pathological age-related changes of the macula, namely drusen maculopathy, geographic atrophy (dry form) and choroidal neovascularization (CNV) (wet or neovascular form). AMD is characterized by a progressive loss of central vision resulting from degenerative and neovascular changes in the macula [5].

Although during the last decade numerous studies were addressed to understand the pathophysiological mechanisms, the underlying processes and modulating factors still need to be elucidated. A growing body of evidence indicates that AMD pathogenesis involves chronic inflammation, complement activation and autoimmunity [6–8].

All subtypes of AMD are complex, multifactorial diseases with only limited means for prevention or cure. Until recently, argon laser photocoagulation and photodynamic therapy (PDT) were the only treatments available for the neovascular form of AMD. The introduction of new intravitreally injectable inhibitors of vascular endothelial growth factor (VEGF) revolutionized the management of the wet form [9, 10].

VEGF is a homodimeric glycoprotein with a molecular weight of 45 kDa which exists in four major isoforms (VEGF-121, -165, -189, -206) [11]. The different isoforms are characterized by their molecular weight, ability to bind to heparin and acidity. VEGF is a key regulator of physiological angiogenesis during embryogenesis but has also been implicated in pathological angiogenesis such as tumor growth or intraocular neovascular diseases [12]. In vivo mouse models demonstrated the impact of VEGF on ocular neovascularization and identified it as a central molecular mediator of CNV, which is the major cause of visual loss in patients with exudative AMD [13]. The binding of VEGF to its receptors on retinal vascular endothelial cells initiates several intracellular signaling pathways resulting in proliferation, differentiation and migration of endothelial cells [14, 15]. In addition, VEGF acts as a potent vascular permeability factor resulting in increased fluid leakage across the blood vessel walls. CNV membranes obtained from patients with AMD contain VEGF as shown in immunohistochemical studies [16, 17]. Analysis of different retinal cell types in post-mortem eyes with AMD revealed higher VEGF levels in the retinal pigment epithelial (RPE) cell layer and the outer nuclear layer than in healthy control eyes [18]. The ability of RPE cells to secrete VEGF has also been shown in in vitro experiments when cells are cultured under hypoxic conditions [19]. Furthermore, significantly increased levels of VEGF have been found in the aqueous humor of human eyes with neovascular AMD as compared to healthy controls [20].

Finally, evidence from clinical trials with anti-VEGF agents in humans, as described below, highlight the pathognomonic role of VEGF in the pathogenesis of neovascular AMD.

Pegaptanib

Pegaptanib, an oligonucleotide aptamer, was the first anti-VEGF agent to be approved by the US Food and Drug Administration (FDA) for use in neovascular AMD. Aptamers are nucleic acid ligands, which bind different targets such as proteins with high specificity and affinity. They are complex three-dimensional structures isolated from oligonucleotides by a selection process in vitro. By binding to molecules, aptamers may change the shape of the molecule or inhibit the molecule's biological function [21–23]. When the anti-VEGF aptamer binds to VEGF it blocks the binding of VEGF to its receptor, preventing the initiation of the intracellular cascade [24]. Pegaptanib consists of a 28-base RNA oligonucleotide with two branched 20-kDa polyethylene glycol moieties, which binds selectively to the VEGF-165 isoform [25].

In August 1998, a phase 1A trial was initiated as a multicenter, open-label, dose-escalation study by the Eyetech Study Group. A total of 15 patients aged between 64 and 92 years with subfoveal CNV secondary to AMD were recruited and received a single injection of pegaptanib at doses between 0.25 and 3.00 mg per eye. Three months after injection, 80% of eyes had an improved or stable vision and 26.7% of eyes showed a significantly improved vision defined as a three-line or greater increase of vision on the ETDRS chart. There were no unexpected visual safety events reported and evaluation of color photographs and fluorescein angiograms showed no signs of choroidal or retinal toxicity [26].

Following the phase 1A trial, a phase 2 study was started to determine the safety profile of a multiple injection therapy. The trial was performed as a multicenter, open-label, repeat-dose study of 3 mg per eye of pegaptanib with and without PDT. 21 patients with subfoveal CNV secondary to AMD were followed up at 11 sites in the USA. Pegaptanib was administered as an intravitreal injection on three occasions at 28-day intervals. PDT with verteporfin was given 5–10 days before administration of the anti-VEGF aptamer in eyes with predominantly classic CNV. There were no serious drug-related adverse events reported 3 months after treatment. 87.5% of patients receiving pegaptanib alone had stabilized or improved vision after 3 months of treatment and 25% of eyes demonstrated a three-line or greater improvement on the ETDRS charts. When combined with PDT, 60% of eyes showed a gain of three lines on the ETDRS charts compared to 2.2% for those eyes treated with PDT alone. 40% of pegaptanib-treated cases were re-treated with PDT at 3 months while this rate increased to 93% in those eyes treated with PDT alone. The phase 2 trial showed that multiple intravitreal injections of pegaptanib were well tolerated and had a positive effect on vision improvement especially in combination with PDT [27].

By 2001, two concurrent, prospective, randomized, double-blind, multicenter, dose-ranging, controlled clinical trials, named VISION (VEGF Inhibition Study in Ocular Neovascularization) were started at 117 sites throughout the world (USA and Canada – Study 1004; other centers worldwide – Study 1003). In total, 1,208 patients 50 years of age or older with subfoveal CNV due to AMD were included. VISION compared three dosages of intravitreal pegaptanib (0.3, 1.0 or 3.0 mg) with sham injections. Injections were given into one eye every 6 weeks over a period of 48 weeks. The primary endpoint was the proportion of patients who had lost fewer than 15 letters of visual acuity (VA) between baseline and week 54. At week 54, 70% of patients randomized to 0.3 mg pegaptanib ($p < 0.001$), 71% of patients assigned to 1.0 mg pegaptanib ($p < 0.001$) and 65% of patients randomized to 3.0 mg pegaptanib ($p = 0.03$) showed a loss of fewer than 15 letters of VA as compared to 55% of patients randomized to sham injections. In addition, fewer patients of the 0.3-mg pegaptanib group required adjunctive PDT – applied at the investigator's discretion – than patients randomized to the sham group, which was an indirect sign of the beneficial effect of the drug. The results for both concurrent trials were similar with both reaching statistical significance between all doses of pegaptanib and the sham injection for the primary endpoint between baseline and week 54 [28]. There was no dose-response relationship between the three different doses of pegaptanib but a higher percentage of patients receiving the 0.3- or 1.0-mg doses lost fewer than 15 letters compared to the 3.0-mg group.

After 54 weeks, patients who had received pegaptanib were re-randomized to either continue therapy or discontinue treatment. Patients who were re-randomized to continue pegaptanib for another year were statistically significantly more likely to maintain stable VA, defined as loss of less than 15 letters, than those who discontinued the drug. However, when the study was analyzed separately (Study 1004 vs. Study 1003), Study 1004 revealed efficacy at 2 years, whereas this was not the case for Study 1003 for any of the active doses at the second year [29].

In summary, the VISION Study showed that patients receiving pegaptanib lost vision in a smaller rate than those treated with conventional care.

Bevacizumab

Bevacizumab is a full-length recombinant humanized monoclonal antibody with a molecular weight of 149 kDa [30, 31]. It binds to and inhibits all isoforms of vascular endothelial growth factor A (VEGF-A) [30]. Unlike ranibizumab it is glycosylated and has an Fc fragment. Bevacizumab is licensed for the intravenous administration for the treatment of malignant solid tumors [32–34] and is available for off-label use in the treatment of AMD-related CNV [34].

Preliminary preclinical studies in primates showed a lack of retinal penetration of an intravitreally injected full-length antibody directed against epithelial growth factor receptor, which had structural similarities with bevacizumab [35]. However, when the commercially available formulation of bevacizumab was used in retinal penetration studies it was clearly shown that it can penetrate the retina and is transported into the photoreceptor outer segments, the retinal pigment epithelium and the choroid [36, 37].

In two small experimental uncontrolled clinical trials performed in the years 2004 and 2005 by the same study group, bevacizumab was used intravenously in patients with neovascular AMD [38, 39]. Improvements in VA and a decrease in macular thickness as assessed by optical coherence tomography (OCT) have been reported from these trials. The drug was well tolerated by the patients and no serious ocular adverse events occurred except that the treatment was associated with elevated blood pressure, which required antihypertensive medication. Geitzenauer et al. [40] compared safety, VA and anatomic outcomes of 2.5 and 5 mg/kg intravenous bevacizumab in patients with neovascular AMD and reported similar improvements of these parameters in both treatment groups. In patients with pigment epithelial detachment secondary to neovascular AMD, systemic bevacizumab therapy proved beneficial in decreasing lesion height and diameter [41].

In order to reduce the risk of systemic side effects the efficacy of intravitreally injected bevacizumab on a patient with neovascular AMD who responded poorly to intravitreal pegaptanib was investigated [42]. Within 1 week, OCT revealed a resolution of subretinal fluid and an improvement in VA in this patient, which was maintained for the following 4 weeks. This encouraging result led to increased interest in the intravitreal application of bevacizumab for the treatment of wet AMD resulting in the initiation of a growing number of clinical trials [43, 44].

A prospective, non-randomized open-label phase 1 dose-escalation study was performed to investigate the safety and tolerability of a single intravitreal injection of bevacizumab at different doses (1.0, 1.5 or 2.0 mg) [45]. Of the 45 patients with AMD and subfoveal CNV, 43 patients completed the study. Twelve weeks after the injection, vision was stabilized or improved and no unfavorable neovascular lesion-macular changes could be observed. A clinical study evaluating the effect of intravitreal bevacizumab on anterior chamber inflammatory activity showed that there was no inflammatory response detectable clinically or by laser flare meter measurement [46].

Growing evidence for the beneficial use of bevacizumab in patients with wet AMD came from a large number of clinical studies describing improvements of VA and a decrease of macular thickness compared to treatment with PDT and/or intravitreal triamcinolone [47, 48]. Numerous retrospective studies have shown beneficial effects of bevacizumab in patients with neovascular AMD. However, results from these trials need to be interpreted with caution, as there are several limitations like retrospective study design, limited number of patients, non-standardized VA testing and a limited-follow-up.

Spaide et al. [49] conducted a retrospective study of 266 eyes of 266 patients with CNV due to AMD over a period of 12 weeks. They reported a VA improvement in 38.8% of patients at the 3-month follow-up visit. Mean central macular thickness decreased by 127 μm from 340 to 213 μm, which was statistically significant [49].

Similar results from a retrospective study were reported by Rich et al. [50]. Three months after the first intravitreal injection of bevacizumab, 44% of patients had at least a three-line improvement of VA together with a decrease in the 1-mm central retinal thickness, which proved to be statistically significant.

An interventional, consecutive, retrospective case series by Avery et al. [51] included 81 eyes of 79 patients receiving intravitreal bevacizumab on a monthly basis until resolution of macular edema, subretinal fluid or pigment epithelium detachment and revealed a median gain of 20 letters at 8 weeks. Mean retinal thickness of the central 1 mm was also statistically significantly decreased.

Although intravitreal bevacizumab seems to be well tolerated in general according to the published data [52], there are several reports about serious ocular inflammation after intravitreal injection [53–57]. A possible explanation for an increased risk of endophthalmitis might be the Fc domain, which is part of bevacizumab but not ranibizumab. This portion of the antibody is known to facilitate immunological processes like phagocyte activation or complement fixation rendering it more susceptible to pro-inflammatory responses. Furthermore, bevacizumab is produced through a cellular pathway by cultures of mammalian ovarian cancer cells, a process associated with glycosylation of proteins with higher immunogenic potential than the non-glycosylated pure proteins obtained by a bacterial pathway as is the case with ranibizumab. Moreover, bevacizumab is produced for intravenous use and therefore undergoes a less strict purification process than drugs primarily intended for intraocular use.

Ranibizumab

Ranibizumab is a recombinant, humanized antibody antigen-binding fragment (F_{ab}) that binds and neutralizes all known active forms of VEGF-A, a protein that is believed to play a critical role in the formation of new blood vessels (fig. 1).

The US FDA approved ranibizumab for treatment of all fluorescein-angiographic subtypes of CNV secondary to AMD. This approval was based on the results of two phase III studies: the MARINA (Minimally Classic/Occult Trial of the Anti-VEGF Antibody Ranibizumab in the Treatment of Neovascular AMD) Study, which compared ranibizumab against sham treatment in patients with minimally classic or occult with no classic CNV secondary to AMD [58], and the ANCHOR (Anti-VEGF Antibody for the Treatment of Predominantly Classic Choroidal Neovascularization in Age-Related Macular Degeneration) Study, which compared ranibizumab against verteporfin PDT in patients with predominantly classic CNV [59]. Verteporfin PDT was selected as the compared treatment in the latter study because it has been shown to slow the progression of vision loss in patients with this typically more aggressive type of lesion [60, 61], and was the standard treatment when this study was initiated. These two studies (described in detail below) were pivotal evaluations of the

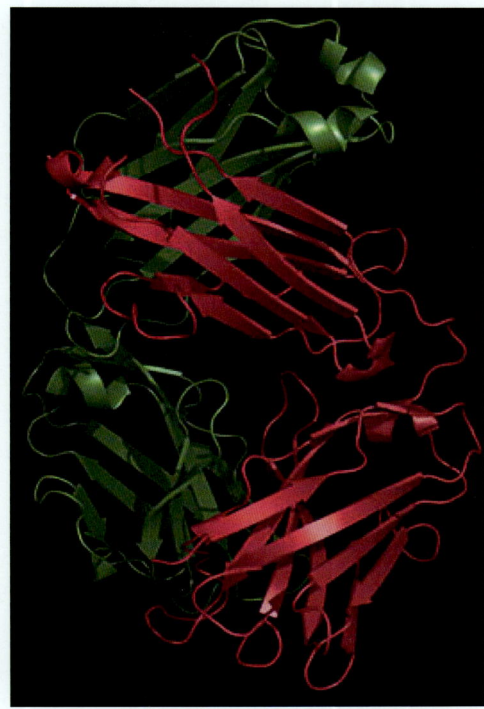

Fig. 1. Ranibizumab (Lucentis®): a humanized monoclonal antibody fragment (F_{ab}) directed against VEGF produced in *Escherichia coli.*

efficacy of ranibizumab and excluded patients who had been previously treated with PDT [62].

A treatment initiation with three consecutive monthly injections, followed by continued monthly injections, has provided the best VA outcomes in pivotal clinical trials. If continued monthly injections are not feasible after initiation, a flexible strategy appears viable, with monthly monitoring of lesion activity recommended. A continuous careful monitoring with flexible retreatment may help avoid recurring vision loss. Still, standardized biomarkers need to be determined. Evidence-based guidelines help to optimize treatment outcomes with ranibizumab in neovascular AMD [63].

A flexible, individualized VA-guided regimen after three initial injections may sustain vision improvement and gives the opportunity to improve the cost-effectiveness and convenience of the treatment and to reduce the incidence of drug administration-associated risks [64]. It has been demonstrated lately that following an initial 3-month loading phase with intravitreal ranibizumab (0.3 mg) the monthly repetition of the intravitreal treatment is clearly superior to injections of 0.3 or 0.5 mg in 3-month intervals in terms of visual-acuity outcome [65].

Although further studies to investigate the risk of stroke with ranibizumab therapy are required, repeated intravitreal ranibizumab is well tolerated and not associated with clinically significant safety risks up to 2 years of treatment [66].

PIER Study

The PIER Study evaluated the efficacy and safety of ranibizumab administered monthly for 3 months and then quarterly in patients with CNV secondary to AMD. Year 1 results were published in October 2007.

This study was a phase IIIb, multicenter, randomized, double-masked, sham injection-controlled trial in patients with predominantly or minimally classic or occult with no classic CNV lesions. Patients were randomized 1:1:1 to 0.3 mg ranibizumab (60 patients), 0.5 mg ranibizumab (61 patients), or sham (63 patients) treatment groups. The primary efficacy endpoint was the mean change from baseline VA at year 1.

Those mean changes from baseline VA were –16.3, –1.6, and –0.2 letters for the sham, 0.3-mg, and 0.5-mg groups, respectively ($p \leq 0.0001$, each ranibizumab dose vs. sham). Ranibizumab stopped growth of the CNV lesions and reduced leakage. However, in the ranibizumab groups the treatment effect declined during quarterly dosing (for example, at 3 months the mean changes from baseline VA had been gains of 2.9 and 4.3 letters for the 0.3- and 0.5-mg doses, respectively). Results of subgroup analyses of mean change from baseline VA at 12 months by baseline age, VA, and lesion characteristics were consistent with the overall results. Few serious ocular or non-ocular adverse events occurred in any group.

The conclusion was that ranibizumab administered monthly for 3 months and then quarterly provided a significant benefit in VA to patients with AMD-related subfoveal CNV and was well tolerated. The incidence of serious ocular or non-ocular adverse events was low [67].

FOCUS Study

The FOCUS Study assessed the efficacy and adverse-events profile of a combined treatment with ranibizumab and verteporfin PDT in patients with predominantly classic CNV secondary to AMD during a 2-year, multicenter, randomized, single-masked, controlled study. The 2-year results were published in December 2007.

106 patients received monthly intravitreal injections of ranibizumab 0.5 mg and 56 patients received sham injections. All patients received PDT on day 0, and then every 3 months as needed. The efficacy assessment included VA changes and changes of the morphology of the lesion and the PDT frequency. Adverse events were summarized by incidence and severity. At the end of year 2, 88% of the patients receiving combined ranibizumab and PDT treatment had lost fewer than 15 letters from baseline VA, whereas 75% of the patients receiving PDT alone had lost fewer than 15 letters. 25% of the patients in the combined treatment group had gained more than 15 letters (7% for the PDT-alone group). The two treatment arms differed by 12.4 letters in mean VA change. The VA benefit of adding ranibizumab to PDT in year 1 persisted through year 2.

On average, patients in the combined treatment group developed less lesion growth and showed greater reduction of CNV leakage and subretinal fluid accumulation, and required fewer PDT retreatments than patients receiving PDT alone (mean 0.4 vs. 3.0 PDT retreatments). Endophthalmitis and serious intraocular inflammation occurred in 2.9% and 12.4% of ranibizumab + PDT patients and 0% of PDT-alone patients. Incidences of serious non-ocular adverse events were similar in the two treatment groups [62].

MARINA Study

In the MARINA (Minimally Classic/Occult Trial of the Anti-VEGF Antibody Ranibizumab in the Treatment of Neovascular AMD) Study, 716 patients with either minimally classic or occult (with no classic lesions) CNV secondary to AMD were randomly assigned to receive 24 monthly intravitreal injections of ranibizumab (either 0.3 or 0.5 mg) or sham injections. The primary endpoint was the proportion of patients losing fewer than 15 letters from baseline VA at 12 months.

At 12 months, 94.5% of the group given 0.3 mg of ranibizumab and 94.6% of those given 0.5 mg had lost fewer than 15 letters, whereas 62.2% of the patients receiving sham injections did so. VA improved by 15 or more letters in 24.8% of the 0.3-mg group and 33.8% of the 0.5-mg group, but only 5.0% of the sham-injection group gained 15 or more letters in VA. Mean increases were 6.5 letters in the 0.3-mg group and 7.2 letters in the 0.5-mg group; the main decrease was 10.4 letters in the sham-injection group. The benefit in VA was maintained at 24 months. During 24 months, presumed endophthalmitis was identified in 5 patients (1.0%) and serious uveitis in 6 patients (1.3%) given ranibizumab.

The study showed that the intravitreal administration of ranibizumab during 2 years did prevent vision loss and improved mean VA and had low rates of serious adverse events, in patients with minimally classic or occult CNV secondary to AMD [58].

ANCHOR Study

The ANCHOR Study (published 2009) demonstrated that ranibizumab was superior to PDT with respect to VA and morphologic efficacy outcomes and that intravitreal treatment of predominantly classic CNV in AMD with ranibizumab had a low rate of serious ocular adverse events.

Of 423 patients (143 PDT, 140 each in the two ranibizumab groups), the majority (77% in each group) completed the 2-year study. At month 24, the VA benefit from ranibizumab was statistically significant (p 0.0001 vs. PDT) and clinically meaningful: 89.9–90.0% of ranibizumab-treated patients had lost fewer than 15 letters from baseline (vs. 65.7% of PDT patients); 34–41.0% had gained 15 or more letters (vs. 6.3% of PDT group). On average, VA had improved from baseline by 8.1–10.7 letters (vs. a mean decline of 9.8 letters in PDT group). Changes in morphological characteristics on FA also favored ranibizumab.

There was no difference among groups in rates of serious ocular and non-ocular adverse events. Three out of 277 patients (1.1%) in the ranibizumab groups developed endophthalmitis in the study eye. Ranibizumab provided greater clinical benefit than verteporfin PDT in patients with AMD with new-onset, predominantly classic CNV.

PrONTO Study

The long-term efficacy of a variable-dosing regimen with ranibizumab was assessed in the 'Prospective Optical Coherence Tomography Imaging of Patients with Neovascular Age-Related Macular Degeneration Treated with Intraocular Ranibizumab' (PrONTO) Study, in which patients were followed for 2 years. The 2-year results were published in January 2009.

The study design was a 2-year prospective, uncontrolled, variable-dosing regimen with intravitreal ranibizumab treatment based on OCT findings. In this open-label, prospective, single-center, uncontrolled clinical study, patients with AMD involving the central fovea and a central retinal thickness of 300 μm or more as measured by OCT received 3 consecutive monthly intravitreal injections of ranibizumab (0.5 mg). During the first year, a retreatment with ranibizumab was performed at each monthly visit if any criterion was fulfilled such as an increase in central retinal thickness of at least 100 μm as assessed by OCT or a loss of 5 letters or more. During the second year, the retreatment criteria were amended to include retreatment if any qualitative increase in the amount of fluid was detected using OCT.

40 patients were enrolled and 37 completed the 2-year study. At month 24, mean VA improved by 11.1 letters ($p < 0.001$) and the OCT-CRT decreased by 212 μm ($p < 0.001$). VA improved by 15 letters or more in 43% of patients. These VA and OCT outcomes were achieved with an average of 9.9 injections over 24 months.

The PrONTO Study using an OCT-guided variable-dosing regimen with intravitreal ranibizumab resulted in VA outcomes comparable with the outcomes from the phase III clinical studies, but fewer intravitreal injections were required [68].

New Anti-VEGF Treatments for Neovascular Age-Related Macular Degeneration

Vascular Endothelial Growth Factor Trap

The VEGF trap is a pharmacologically engineered protein that binds VEGF and thus prevents VEGF binding to its cellular receptor. The VEGF trap is composed of two different binding domains from VEGF receptor 1 and 2, and is designed to bind the VEGF-A isoform with higher affinity than pegaptanib or ranibizumab to offer a theoretically longer interval between necessary treatments [69].

The intravitreal VEGF trap has been evaluated in a phase 1/2 study, the Clinical Evaluation of Anti-Angiogenesis in the Retina (CLEAR)-IT 1 and 2. 21 participants with neovascular AMD were treated with a single intravitreal dose (0.05, 0.15, 0.5, 1, 2, or 4 mg) of the VEGF trap. In the two highest dose groups (2 and 4 mg), the mean increase in best corrected VA was 13.5 letters. In addition, the mean time for retreatment was 150 days (range 45–420). No serious ocular or systemic adverse events were noted [70].

Combined Therapy Regiments

The effect of combined treatment of CNV secondary to AMD is subject to actual research. The pro-angiogenic and pro-inflammatory effects of verteporfin could be counteracted by combined treatment with anti-VEGF agents [71]. During a single-center, prospective clinical study conducted at the Department of Ophthalmology of the Medical University of Vienna, the combined treatment with verteporfin/ranibizumab was associated with CNV occlusion, reduced edema, improved visual function and retinal sensitivity [72]. Same-day verteporfin and ranibizumab appears to be safe and is not associated with severe vision loss or severe ocular inflammation [73].

Imaging Anti-VEGF Effects on Retinal Morphology in Age-Related Macular Degeneration

During recent years, OCT has emerged as an important tool in the diagnosis of AMD and during the follow-up period following anti-VEGF treatment [74]. OCT allows a detailed evaluation of retinal morphology, similar to in vivo histology, providing insights into characteristic in vivo changes that occur during disease progression as well as secondary to treatment. The fourth-generation OCT, spectral-domain OCT (SD-OCT), uses a fast spectral domain technique and performs scans in a raster pattern throughout the entire macular area at a very high resolution [75, 76] (fig. 2).

The fifth-generation OCT, the polarization sensitive OCT (PS-OCT), enables to detect retinal tissue due to its different qualities of polarization and allows specifically the detection of RPE cells [77, 78]. The combination of PS-SD-OCT provides a precise identification of retinal pigment epithelium in AMD, allowing the recognition of disease-specific patterns in order to identify the status and progression of AMD [79].

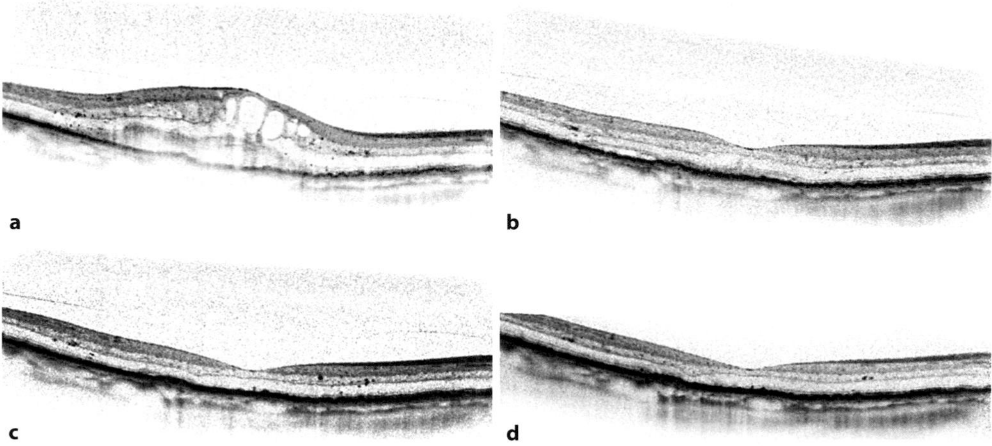

Fig. 2. SD-OCT images taken of a patient with CNV secondary to AMD: (**a**) at baseline, (**b**) month 1 follow-up of the same patient, (**c**) month 3 follow-up, and (**d**) month 6 follow-up.

High-definition images of the retina obtained by SD-OCT visualize the effect of VEGF inhibition on retinal morphology over time in detail [80, 81]. A precise understanding of morphological changes of different retinal and subretinal layers under anti-VEGF therapy is crucial for the identification of parameters relevant for functional improvement and prognosis [47, 82–84].

Several clinical studies investigated morphological and functional effects of intravitreally applied ranibizumab in patients with CNV secondary to AMD. OCT data from the MARINA, Safety Assessment of Intravitreal Lucentis for AMD (SAILOR), PIER, and PrONTO studies showed that within days after injection of ranibizumab, stabilized or improved VA was accompanied by a decrease in macular thickness and reduction of leakage of intra- and subretinal fluid [85–89].

OCT allows the quantitative determination of efficacy and potential effective duration of action of a therapeutic agent in a non-invasive and simple manner. Shah and Del Priore [90] used sequential OCT measurements to determine the magnitude and time course of the initial response to anti-VEGF treatment and the subsequent return of exudation after single and multiple intravitreal injections of bevacizumab and ranibizumab in eyes with no prior anti-VEGF treatment. Both drugs proved equally effective at reducing central foveal thickness or macular volume. However, it took longer for bevacizumab to achieve the minimum macular volume and its effects took longer to wear off.

Witkin et al. [91] showed that the reduction in retinal thickness 1 month after anti-VEGF injection is primarily the result of reduction in permeability in the neovascular lesion, followed by a reduction in intra- and subretinal fluid, without reduction in the size of the CNV lesion.

Size and location of the CNV lesion in relation to the RPE level were qualitatively and quantitatively determined two-dimensionally by Fremme et al. [92], in order to get an impression of classic and occult CNV components. The authors reported that under ranibizumab monotherapy there was no clinically significant regression of CNV.

In a prospective study, Bolz et al. [93] identified and quantified the effects of intravitreal ranibizumab therapy given as a loading regimen with three injections during the first 3 months with Stratus OCT. Significant morphological and functional therapeutic effects were observed as early as 1 week following the first treatment with ranibizumab. During the loading-dose period, central retinal thickness, intraretinal cysts and subretinal fluid decreased fast and significantly, whereas pigment epithelial detachment resolved less rapidly. The initial administration of intravitreal ranibizumab induced a significant effect on intra- and subretinal fluid and visual function; subsequent injections had a less pronounced effect. The change in morphology and function was only significant between baseline and week 1, while there were no significant additional morphological or functional benefits following the second and third injection.

Similar results were reported from Ahlers et al. [94] in a prospective case series analyzing the effect of 3-monthly doses of ranibizumab on retinal morphology and visual outcome in patients with AMD. The study showed that the central millimeter thickness of the retina as measured by Stratus OCT significantly decreased within the first week after initial ranibizumab treatment. Most of the maximal therapeutic effect was obtained within this time period. A further decrease in retinal thickness could be observed continuously up to month 3. Furthermore, OCT revealed that subretinal fluid was reduced 1 week after the first injection and was almost eliminated 1 month later. Over the period of the next 2 months, no additional major changes could be observed. Pigment epithelial detachment was also significantly reduced within the first week after the initial treatment with a continuous resolution over the next 3 months. Furthermore, the study showed that a reduction of retinal thickness correlated with an improvement in BCVA. The same could be demonstrated for the decrease in subretinal fluid, which correlated significantly with an improvement in BCVA. In contrast, there was no significant correlation between pigment epithelial detachment and VA. Overall, the best therapeutic effect of VA improvement was observed 1 month after the first injection of ranibizumab suggesting that morphological recovery occurred at an earlier timepoint than visual improvement. In a similar study design, Kiss et al. [95] evaluated the effect of three injections of ranibizumab on retinal function and morphology in 23 patients affected by neovascular AMD. The results of the study suggest that the RPE lesion area may be more relevant for visual function than retinal thickness.

Apart from a morphological benefit, there are case reports describing RPE tears following anti-VEGF therapy. RPE tears may occur after intravitreal injection of ranibizumab in patients with neovascular AMD, probably because of the rapid regression of the fibrovascular membrane [96, 97]. A small ratio of CNV size to pigment epithelial detachment is more common in eyes with RPE tears. In addition, a larger size of pigment epithelial detachment is considered as a predictor for RPE tears. However, vision may be preserved despite RPE tears [98]. Although a pigment epithelial tear in neovascular AMD can represent natural history, it is suggested that clinicians should be aware of and monitor patients for the possibility of this complication after intravitreal injections of ranibizumab [99]. However, it remains to be determined if a pigment epithelial tear should be considered as a possible therapeutically induced complication or if it rather represents natural history in neovascular AMD.

In summary, a number of studies have shown that OCT imaging allows identification of functionally relevant factors like subretinal fluid or retinal thickness, which are important for the establishment of an optimized individual dosing regimen during antiangiogenesis therapies.

References

1 VanNewkirk MR, Nanjan MB, Wang JJ, et al: The prevalence of age-related maculopathy: the visual impairment project. Ophthalmology 2000;107:1593–1600.
2 Mitchell P, Smith W, Attebo K, Wang JJ: Prevalence of age-related maculopathy in Australia. The Blue Mountains Eye Study. Ophthalmology 1995;102:1450–1460.
3 Buch H, Nielsen NV, Vinding T, et al: Fourteen-year incidence, progression, and visual morbidity of age-related maculopathy: the Copenhagen City Eye Study. Ophthalmology 2005;112:787–798.
4 Klein R, Klein BE, Knudtson MD, et al: Fifteen-year cumulative incidence of age-related macular degeneration: the Beaver Dam Eye Study. Ophthalmology 2007;114:253–262.
5 Witmer AN, Vrensen GF, Van Noorden CJ, Schlingemann RO: Vascular endothelial growth factors and angiogenesis in eye disease. Prog Retin Eye Res 2003;22:1–29.
6 Reynolds R, Hartnett ME, Atkinson JP, et al: Plasma complement components and activation fragments: associations with age-related macular degeneration genotypes and phenotypes. Invest Ophthalmol Vis Sci 2009;50:5818–5827.
7 Morohoshi K, Goodwin AM, Ohbayashi M, Ono SJ: Autoimmunity in retinal degeneration: autoimmune retinopathy and age-related macular degeneration. J Autoimmun 2009;33:247–254.
8 Okemefuna AI, Nan R, Miller A, et al: Complement factor H binds at two independent sites to C-reactive protein in acute phase concentrations. J Biol Chem 2010;285:1053–1065.
9 Schmidt-Erfurth U, Pruente C: Management of neovascular age-related macular degeneration. Prog Retin Eye Res 2007;26:437–451.
10 Schmidt-Erfurth U, Richard G, Augustin A, et al: Guidance for the treatment of neovascular age-related macular degeneration. Acta Ophthalmol Scand 2007;85:486–494.
11 Ferrara N, Gerber HP, LeCouter J: The biology of VEGF and its receptors. Nat Med 2003;9:669–676.
12 Carmeliet P: Mechanisms of angiogenesis and arteriogenesis. Nat Med 2000;6:389–395.
13 Ishibashi T, Hata Y, Yoshikawa H, et al: Expression of vascular endothelial growth factor in experimental choroidal neovascularization. Graefes Arch Clin Exp Ophthalmol 1997;235:159–167.
14 Kvanta A: Ocular angiogenesis: the role of growth factors. Acta Ophthalmol Scand 2006;84:282–288.
15 Petrova TV, Makinen T, Alitalo K: Signaling via vascular endothelial growth factor receptors. Exp Cell Res 1999;253:117–130.
16 Frank RN, Amin RH, Eliott D, et al: Basic fibroblast growth factor and vascular endothelial growth factor are present in epiretinal and choroidal neovascular membranes. Am J Ophthalmol 1996;122:393–403.

17 Kvanta A, Algvere PV, Berglin L, Seregard S: Subfoveal fibrovascular membranes in age-related macular degeneration express vascular endothelial growth factor. Invest Ophthalmol Vis Sci 1996;37: 1929–1934.
18 Kliffen M, Sharma HS, Mooy CM, et al: Increased expression of angiogenic growth factors in age-related maculopathy. Br J Ophthalmol 1997;81:154–162.
19 Shima DT, Adamis AP, Ferrara N, et al: Hypoxic induction of endothelial cell growth factors in retinal cells: identification and characterization of vascular endothelial growth factor as the mitogen. Mol Med 1995;1:182–193.
20 Funk M, Karl D, Georgopoulos M, et al: Neovascular age-related macular degeneration: intraocular cytokines and growth factors and the influence of therapy with ranibizumab. Ophthalmology 2009; 116:2393–2399.
21 Waheed NK, Miller JW: Aptamers, intramers, and vascular endothelial growth factor. Int Ophthalmol Clin 2004;44:11–22.
22 Famulok M, Mayer G, Blind M: Nucleic acid aptamers – from selection in vitro to applications in vivo. Acc Chem Res 2000;33:591–599.
23 Ellington AD, Szostak JW: In vitro selection of RNA molecules that bind specific ligands. Nature 1990;346:818–822.
24 Schachat AP: New treatments for age-related macular degeneration. Ophthalmology 2005;112:531–532.
25 Ruckman J, Green LS, Beeson J, et al: 2′-Fluoropyrimidine RNA-based aptamers to the 165-amino-acid form of vascular endothelial growth factor (VEGF-165). Inhibition of receptor binding and VEGF-induced vascular permeability through interactions requiring the exon 7 encoded domain. J Biol Chem 1998;273:20556–20567.
26 Eyetech Study Group: Preclinical and phase 1A clinical evaluation of an anti-VEGF pegylated aptamer (EYE001) for the treatment of exudative age-related macular degeneration. Retina 2002;22:143–152.
27 Eyetech Study Group: Anti-vascular endothelial growth factor therapy for subfoveal choroidal neovascularization secondary to age-related macular degeneration: phase II study results. Ophthalmology 2003;110:979–986.
28 Gragoudas ES, Adamis AP, Cunningham ET Jr, et al: Pegaptanib for neovascular age-related macular degeneration. N Engl J Med 2004;351:2805–2816.
29 Spaide R: New treatments for AMD. Ophthalmology 2006;113:160–161.
30 Ferrara N, Hillan KJ, Gerber HP, Novotny W: Discovery and development of bevacizumab, an anti-VEGF antibody for treating cancer. Nat Rev Drug Discov 2004;3:391–400.
31 Presta LG, Chen H, O'Connor SJ, et al: Humanization of an anti-vascular endothelial growth factor monoclonal antibody for the therapy of solid tumors and other disorders. Cancer Res 1997;57:4593–4599.
32 Adding a humanized antibody to vascular endothelial growth factor (bevacizumab, Avastin) to chemotherapy improves survival in metastatic colorectal cancer. Clin Colorectal Cancer 2003;3:85–88.
33 Kabbinavar F, Hurwitz HI, Fehrenbacher L, et al: Phase II, randomized trial comparing bevacizumab plus fluorouracil (FU)/leucovorin (LV) with FU/LV alone in patients with metastatic colorectal cancer. J Clin Oncol 2003;21:60–65.
34 Hurwitz H, Fehrenbacher L, Novotny W, et al: Bevacizumab plus irinotecan, fluorouracil, and leucovorin for metastatic colorectal cancer. N Engl J Med 2004;350:2335–2342.
35 Mordenti J, Cuthbertson RA, Ferrara N, et al: Comparisons of the intraocular tissue distribution, pharmacokinetics, and safety of ^{125}I-labeled full-length and F_{ab} antibodies in rhesus monkeys following intravitreal administration. Toxicol Pathol 1999; 27:536–544.
36 Heiduschka P, Fietz H, Hofmeister S, et al: Penetration of bevacizumab through the retina after intravitreal injection in the monkey. Invest Ophthalmol Vis Sci 2007;48:2814–2823.
37 Shahar J, Avery RL, Heilweil G, et al: Electrophysiologic and retinal penetration studies following intravitreal injection of bevacizumab (Avastin). Retina 2006;26:262–269.
38 Michels S, Rosenfeld PJ, Puliafito CA, et al: Systemic bevacizumab (Avastin) therapy for neovascular age-related macular degeneration 12-week results of an uncontrolled open-label clinical study. Ophthalmology 2005;112:1035–1047.
39 Moshfeghi AA, Rosenfeld PJ, Puliafito CA, et al: Systemic bevacizumab (Avastin) therapy for neovascular age-related macular degeneration: 24-week results of an uncontrolled open-label clinical study. Ophthalmology 2006;113:2002.e1–12.
40 Geitzenauer W, Michels S, Prager F, et al: Comparison of 2.5 and 5 mg/kg systemic bevacizumab in neovascular age-related macular degeneration: 24-week results of an uncontrolled, prospective cohort study. Retina 2008;28:1375–1386.
41 Bolz M, Michels S, Geitzenauer W, et al: Effect of systemic bevacizumab therapy on retinal pigment epithelial detachment. Br J Ophthalmol 2007;91: 785–789.
42 Rosenfeld PJ, Fung AE, Puliafito CA: Optical coherence tomography findings after an intravitreal injection of bevacizumab (Avastin) for macular edema from central retinal vein occlusion. Ophthalmic Surg Lasers Imaging 2005;36:336–339.

43 Weigert G, Michels S, Sacu S, et al: Intravitreal bevacizumab (Avastin) therapy versus photodynamic therapy plus intravitreal triamcinolone for neovascular age-related macular degeneration: 6-month results of a prospective, randomised, controlled clinical study. Br J Ophthalmol 2008;92:356–360.
44 Hahn R, Sacu S, Michels S, et al: Intravitreal bevacizumab versus verteporfin and intravitreal triamcinolone acetonide in patients with neovascular age-related macula degeneration (in German). Ophthalmologe 2007;104:588–593.
45 Costa RA, Jorge R, Calucci D, et al: Intravitreal bevacizumab for choroidal neovascularization caused by AMD (IBeNA Study): results of a phase 1 dose-escalation study. Invest Ophthalmol Vis Sci 2006; 47:4569–4578.
46 Kiss C, Michels S, Prager F, et al: Evaluation of anterior chamber inflammatory activity in eyes treated with intravitreal bevacizumab. Retina 2006;26:877–881.
47 Leydolt C, Michels S, Prager F, et al: Effect of intravitreal bevacizumab (Avastin®) in neovascular age-related macular degeneration using a treatment regimen based on optical coherence tomography: 6- and 12-month results. Acta Ophthalmol 2009: [Epub ahead of print].
48 Sacu S, Michels S, Prager F, et al: Randomised clinical trial of intravitreal Avastin vs. photodynamic therapy and intravitreal triamcinolone: long-term results. Eye (Lond) 2009;23:2223–2227.
49 Spaide RF, Laud K, Fine HF, et al: Intravitreal bevacizumab treatment of choroidal neovascularization secondary to age-related macular degeneration. Retina 2006;26:383–390.
50 Rich RM, Rosenfeld PJ, Puliafito CA, et al: Short-term safety and efficacy of intravitreal bevacizumab (Avastin) for neovascular age-related macular degeneration. Retina 2006;26:495–511.
51 Avery RL, Pieramici DJ, Rabena MD, et al: Intravitreal bevacizumab (Avastin) for neovascular age-related macular degeneration. Ophthalmology 2006;113:363–372.e5.
52 Fung AE, Rosenfeld PJ, Reichel E: The International Intravitreal Bevacizumab Safety Survey: using the internet to assess drug safety worldwide. Br J Ophthalmol 2006;90:1344–1349.
53 Artunay O, Yuzbasioglu E, Rasier R, et al: Incidence and management of acute endophthalmitis after intravitreal bevacizumab (Avastin) injection. Eye (Lond) 2009;23:2187–2193.
54 Sato T, Emi K, Ikeda T, et al: Severe intraocular inflammation after intravitreal injection of bevacizumab. Ophthalmology 2010;117:512–516.e1–2.
55 Yenerel NM, Dinc UA, Gorgun E: A case of sterile endophthalmitis after repeated intravitreal bevacizumab injection. J Ocul Pharmacol Ther 2008;24: 362–363.
56 Yamashiro K, Tsujikawa A, Miyamoto K, et al: Sterile endophthalmitis after intravitreal injection of bevacizumab obtained from a single batch. Retina 2010;30:485–490.
57 Georgopoulos M, Polak K, Prager F, et al: Characteristics of severe intraocular inflammation following intravitreal injection of bevacizumab (Avastin). Br J Ophthalmol 2009;93:457–462.
58 Rosenfeld PJ, Brown DM, Heier JS, et al: Ranibizumab for neovascular age-related macular degeneration. N Engl J Med 2006;355:1419–1431.
59 Brown DM, Kaiser PK, Michels M, et al: Ranibizumab versus verteporfin for neovascular age-related macular degeneration. N Engl J Med 2006; 355:1432–1444.
60 TAP Report 1: Photodynamic therapy of subfoveal choroidal neovascularization in age-related macular degeneration with verteporfin: one-year results of two randomized clinical trials. Arch Ophthalmol 1999;117:1329–1345.
61 TAP Report 2: Photodynamic therapy of subfoveal choroidal neovascularization in age-related macular degeneration with verteporfin: two-year results of two randomized clinical trials. Arch Ophthalmol 2001;119:198–207.
62 Andrew NA, Lisa T, Carol YC, Angele S: Ranibizumab combined with verteporfin photodynamic therapy in neovascular age-related macular degeneration (FOCUS): year 2 results. Am J Ophthalmol 2008;145:862–874.e3.
63 Mitchell P, Korobelnik JF, Lanzetta P, et al: Ranibizumab (Lucentis) in neovascular age-related macular degeneration: evidence from clinical trials. Br J Ophthalmol 2009;20:20.
64 Holz FG, Korobelnik JF, Lanzetta P, et al: The effects of a flexible visual acuity-driven ranibizumab treatment regimen in age-related macular degeneration: outcomes of a drug and disease model. Invest Ophthalmol Vis Sci 2009;51:405–412.
65 Schmidt-Erfurth U, Eldem B, Guymer R, et al.; on behalf of the EXCITE Study Group: Efficacy and safety of monthly versus quarterly ranibizumab treatment in neovascular age-related macular degeneration. Ophthalmology 2010 (in press).
66 Schmidt-Erfurth U: Clinical safety of ranibizumab in age-related macular degeneration. Expert Opin Drug Saf 2010;9:149–165.
67 Carl DR, David MB, Prema A, et al: Randomized, double-masked, sham-controlled trial of ranibizumab for neovascular age-related macular degeneration: PIER Study year 1. Am J Ophthalmol 2008;145:239–248.e5.

68 Lalwani GA, Rosenfeld PJ, Fung AE, et al: A variable-dosing regimen with intravitreal ranibizumab for neovascular age-related macular degeneration: year 2 of the PrONTO Study. Am J Ophthalmol 2009;148:43–58.e1.
69 Quan Dong N, Syed Mahmood S, Gulnar H, et al: A phase I trial of an IV-administered vascular endothelial growth factor trap for treatment in patients with choroidal neovascularization due to age-related macular degeneration. Ophthalmology 2006;113:1522.e1–14.
70 Do DV: Antiangiogenic approaches to age-related macular degeneration in the future. Ophthalmology 2009;116(suppl 1):S24–S6.
71 Schmidt-Erfurth U, Schlotzer-Schrehard U, Cursiefen C, et al: Influence of photodynamic therapy on expression of vascular endothelial growth factor (VEGF), VEGF receptor 3, and pigment epithelium-derived factor. Invest Ophthalmol Vis Sci 2003;44:4473–4480.
72 Kiss CG, Simader C, Michels S, Schmidt-Erfurth U: Combination of verteporfin photodynamic therapy and ranibizumab: effects on retinal anatomy, choroidal perfusion and visual function in the protect study. Br J Ophthalmol 2008;92:1620–1627.
73 Schmidt-Erfurth U, Wolf S: Same-day administration of verteporfin and ranibizumab 0.5 mg in patients with choroidal neovascularisation due to age-related macular degeneration. Br J Ophthalmol 2008;92:1628–1635.
74 Srinivasan VJ, Wojtkowski M, Witkin AJ, et al: High-definition and three-dimensional imaging of macular pathologies with high-speed ultrahigh-resolution optical coherence tomography. Ophthalmology 2006;113:2054.e1–14.
75 Golbaz I, Ahlers C, Goesseringer N, et al: Automatic and manual segmentation of healthy retinas using high-definition optical coherence tomography. Acta Ophthalmol 2009: [Epub ahead of print].
76 Mylonas G, Ahlers C, Malamos P, et al: Comparison of retinal thickness measurements and segmentation performance of four different spectral and time domain OCT devices in neovascular age-related macular degeneration. Br J Ophthalmol 2009;93:1453–1460.
77 Gotzinger E, Pircher M, Baumann B, et al: Three-dimensional polarization sensitive OCT imaging and interactive display of the human retina. Opt Express 2009;17:4151–4165.
78 Ahlers C, Schmidt-Erfurth U: Three-dimensional high resolution OCT imaging of macular pathology. Opt Express 2009;17:4037–4045.
79 Ahlers C, Gotzinger E, Pircher M, et al: Imaging of the retinal pigment epithelium in age-related macular degeneration using polarization-sensitive optical coherence tomography. Invest Ophthalmol Vis Sci 2010;51:2149–2157.
80 Puliafito CA, Hee MR, Lin CP, et al: Imaging of macular diseases with optical coherence tomography. Ophthalmology 1995;102:217–229.
81 Pieroni CG, Witkin AJ, Ko TH, et al: Ultrahigh resolution optical coherence tomography in non-exudative age-related macular degeneration. Br J Ophthalmol 2006;90:191–197.
82 Malamos P, Sacu S, Georgopoulos M, et al: Correlation of high-definition optical coherence tomography and fluorescein angiography imaging in neovascular macular degeneration. Invest Ophthalmol Vis Sci 2009;50:4926–4933.
83 Golbaz I, Ahlers C, Schutze C, et al: Influence of antiangiogenetic therapy on retinal thickness values in age-related macular degeneration (in German). Ophthalmologe 2009;106:1103–1110.
84 Einwallner E, Ahlers C, Golbaz I, et al: Neovascular age-related macular degeneration under anti-angiogenic therapy: subretinal fluid is a relevant prognostic parameter (in German). Ophthalmologe 2010;107:158–164.
85 Andreoli CM, Miller JW: Antivascular endothelial growth factor therapy for ocular neovascular disease. Curr Opin Ophthalmol 2007;18:502–508.
86 Brown DM, Regillo CD: Anti-VEGF agents in the treatment of neovascular age-related macular degeneration: applying clinical trial results to the treatment of everyday patients. Am J Ophthalmol 2007;144:627–637.
87 Brown DM, Kaiser PK, Michels M, et al: Ranibizumab versus verteporfin for neovascular age-related macular degeneration. N Engl J Med 2006;355:1432–1444.
88 Kaiser PK, Blodi BA, Shapiro H, Acharya NR: Angiographic and optical coherence tomographic results of the MARINA Study of ranibizumab in neovascular age-related macular degeneration. Ophthalmology 2007;114:1868–1875.
89 Regillo CD, Brown DM, Abraham P, et al: Randomized, double-masked, sham-controlled trial of ranibizumab for neovascular age-related macular degeneration: PIER Study year 1. Am J Ophthalmol 2008;145:239–248.
90 Shah AR, Del Priore LV: Duration of action of intravitreal ranibizumab and bevacizumab in exudative AMD eyes based on macular volume measurements. Br J Ophthalmol 2009;93:1027–1032.

91 Witkin AJ, Vuong LN, Srinivasan VJ, et al: High-speed ultrahigh resolution optical coherence tomography before and after ranibizumab for age-related macular degeneration. Ophthalmology 2009;116:956–963.
92 Framme C, Panagakis G, Birngruber R: Effects on choroidal neovascularization after anti-VEGF upload using intravitreal ranibizumab, as determined by spectral domain-optical coherence tomography. Invest Ophthalmol Vis Sci 2010;51:1671–1676.
93 Bolz M, Simader C, Ritter M, et al: Morphological and functional analysis of the loading regimen with intravitreal ranibizumab in neovascular age-related macular degeneration. Br J Ophthalmol 2010;94:185–189.
94 Ahlers C, Golbaz I, Stock G, et al: Time course of morphologic effects on different retinal compartments after ranibizumab therapy in age-related macular degeneration. Ophthalmology 2008;115:e39–e46.
95 Kiss CG, Geitzenauer W, Simader C, et al: Evaluation of ranibizumab-induced changes in high-resolution optical coherence tomographic retinal morphology and their impact on visual function. Invest Ophthalmol Vis Sci 2009;50:2376–2383.
96 Bakri SJ, Kitzmann AS: Retinal pigment epithelial tear after intravitreal ranibizumab. Am J Ophthalmol 2007;143:505–507.
97 Kiss C, Michels S, Prager F, et al: Retinal pigment epithelium tears following intravitreal ranibizumab therapy. Acta Ophthalmol Scand 2007;85:902–903.
98 Chan CKM, Meyer CHM, et al: Retinal pigment epithelial tears after intravitreal bevacizumab injection for neovascular age-related macular degeneration. Retina 2007;27:541–551.
99 Apte RS: Retinal pigment epithelial tear after intravitreal ranibizumab for subfoveal CNV secondary to AMD. Int Ophthalmol 2007;27:59–61.

Prof. Ursula Schmidt-Erfurth
Department of Ophthalmology and Optometry
Medical University Vienna
Waehringer Guertel 18-20, AT–1090 Vienna (Austria)
E-Mail ursula.schmidt-erfurth@meduniwien.ac.at

Bandello F, Battaglia Parodi M (eds): Anti-VEGF.
Dev Ophthalmol. Basel, Karger, 2010, vol 46, pp 39–53

Antivascular Endothelial Growth Factor in Diabetic Retinopathy

Pierluigi Iacono[a] · Maurizio Battaglia Parodi[b] · Francesco Bandello[b]

[a]Fondazione G.B. Bietti per l'Oftalmologia, IRCCS (Istituto di Ricovero e Cura a Carattere Scientifico), Rome, and [b]Department of Ophthalmology, University Vita-Salute, Scientific Institute San Raffaele, Milan, Italy

Abstract

Diabetic macular edema (DME) and proliferative diabetic retinopathy (PDR) represent the most common causes of vision loss in patients affected by diabetes mellitus. Diabetic retinopathy (DR) needs special attention because of its high public health impact and impact on quality of life of patients. Actually, laser retinal photocoagulation is the standard of care for the treatment of DR. However, laser treatment reduces the risk of moderate visual loss by approximately 50%, without a remarkable vision recovery. Thus, new approaches in the treatment of DR have been taken into account and, more specifically, the therapy employing antivascular endothelial growth factor (anti-VEGF) drugs could play a meaningful role. VEGF is a pluripotent growth factor that functions as an endothelial cell-specific mitogen and vasopermeability factor. Through these mechanisms VEGF plays a critical role in promoting angiogenesis and vascular leakage. A high level of VEGF has been detected in eyes presenting DME and PDR, and thereby VEGF is an attractive candidate as therapeutic target of pharmacological treatment in the management of DR. In the current chapter, the concepts and results of anti-VEGF therapy in the treatment of the DME and PDR are presented.

Diabetic retinopathy (DR) is considered the most frequent vascular disorder being detectable in about 40% of diabetic patients 40 years and older [1]. Today, DR is the leading cause of acquired blindness among young adults throughout the developed countries [2]. Population-based epidemiological studies have estimated that after 20 years, DR is recognized to a certain extent, and that after 30 years a proliferative DR is present in the 70% of patients with diabetes mellitus type 1 [3]. The World Health Organization estimates that about 171 million persons are affected by diabetes with an expected doubling of prevalence expected in the next 20 years [4].

Role of the Vascular Endothelial Growth Factor in Diabetic Retinopathy

Hyperglycemia is the main factor involved in the pathogenesis of DR. It results in the production of glycation end products, activation of the polyol pathway, and altered transduction of cellular signals [5–7]. The following damage to endothelial cells and pericytes, through activation of oxidative and inflammatory mechanisms, produces diabetic microangiopathy affecting small-caliber retinal vessel [8]. These alterations result in the deregulation of the mechanism of flow control with subsequently hypoxia and accumulation of fluid in the retinal tissue. Hypoxia represents the likely major inducer of vascular endothelial growth factor (VEGF) gene transcription, but the overexpression of VEGF is also upregulated in response to high glucose, protein kinase C activation, and glycation end products, all elements characterizing the impairment of glycometabolic control [5–7, 9].

VEGF is a pluripotent growth factor that functions as an endothelial cell-specific mitogen and vasopermeability factor and through these mechanisms the VEGF plays a critical role in promoting angiogenesis and vascular leakage [10–13]. In DR, the impairment of the blood retinal barrier and the increased permeability are responsible for the diabetic macular edema (DME) and several investigations underline the active role of VEGF. By disrupting the intercellular tight junctions between the retinal endothelial cells, VEGF increases the extracellular accumulation of fluid from the intravascular compartment [8]. Moreover, VEGF shows a role in mediating active intraocular neovascularization.

Elevations of VEGF levels in ocular fluids from human patients with tissue hypoxia and active neovascularization secondary to DR have been well documented [14]. The increased levels of VEGF decline when treatment with panretinal photocoagulation induces regression of neovascularization. Thus, these studies demonstrated a temporal correlation between VEGF elevations and active proliferative retinopathy evidencing the role of VEGF as a key mediator of intraocular neovascularization secondary to DR. In essence, VEGF is an attractive candidate as therapeutic target of pharmacological treatment in the management of DR.

Anti-VEGF Therapy in the Treatment of Diabetic Macular Edema and Proliferative Diabetic Retinopathy

The VEGF molecular family includes five members: placental growth factor, VEGF-A, VEGF-B, VEGF-C and VEGF-D [15]. Each of the different factors may link one or more of three VEGF receptors. Moreover, between the different factors, VEGF-A plays a major role in angiogenesis and vascular permeability. Alternative splicing of VEGF gene produces nine VEGF-A isoforms ($VEGF_{121}$, $VEGF_{145}$, $VEGF_{148}$, $VEGF_{162}$, $VEGF_{165}$, $VEGF_{165b}$, $VEGF_{183}$, $VEGF_{189}$, $VEGF_{206}$) and among them $VEGF_{165}$ is the most abundantly expressed isoform and is detected as being mainly responsible for DR.

The pathway enclosed between VEGF gene transcription and the activation of the VEGF receptor is the object of a new therapeutic approach based on the use of the VEGF antagonist. Pegaptanib, ranibizumab, bevacizumab and VEGF Trap are molecules that are able to directly bind the VEGF protein. A new and interesting therapeutic approach is the employment of bevasiranib. This molecule, interfering with messenger RNA, interrupts the synthesis of the VEGF protein. Last of all, rapamycin, employed commonly as an immunosuppressive, anti-inflammatory or antimycotic drug, reduces the activity of VEGF molecules interfering with the promoting signal, the active synthesis of VEGF, and reduces the response of endothelial cells to VEGF.

Ranibizumab

Ranibizumab is an antigen-binding fragment (F_{ab}) derived from a humanized anti-VEGF antibody and this F_{ab} inhibits all biologically active isoforms and active proteolytic fragments of VEGF-A. Currently, ranibizumab is approved by the Food and Drug Administration for the treatment of neovascular age-related macular degeneration.

Chun et al. [16] reported the first pilot study exploring the effects of two dosing regimens of ranibizumab in eyes affected by clinically significant DME. Of 10 patients enrolled, 5 received 0.3 mg ranibizumab and 5 received 0.5 mg ranibizumab at baseline and at 1 and 2 months. At month 3, 40% of patients gained more than 15 letters, 50% gained more than 10 letters, and 80% obtained an improvement of at least 1 letter in best corrected visual acuity (BCVA). At month 3, the mean decrease in central retinal thickness was 45.3 and 197.8 μm in the low- and high-dose groups, respectively. Intravitreal injections of ranibizumab were generally well tolerated and no systemic adverse events were reported.

Nguyen et al. [17] investigated the role of ranibizumab in DME in the open-label study READ-1 (Ranibizumab for Edema of the Macula in Diabetes: Phase 1). Ten patients with chronic DME received intraocular injections of 0.5 mg ranibizumab at baseline and at 1, 2, 4, and 6 months. The main outcome measures were changes in BCVA, central retinal thickness as assessed by optical coherence tomography (OCT) measurement at the 7-month examination. Mean and median values of BCVA improved at 7 months by 12.3 and 11 letters respectively. Compared to the baseline, mean foveal thickness showed a meaningful reduction decreasing from 503 to 257 μm with a 85% reduction of the excess foveal thickness present at baseline. The injections were well tolerated with no ocular or systemic adverse events.

More recently, the results of the READ-2 study were reported. READ-2 was a prospective, randomized, interventional, multicenter clinical trial designed to compare ranibizumab with focal/grid laser, alone or in combination, in DME [18]. 126 patients were randomized to receive 0.5 mg ranibizumab, focal/grid laser photocoagulation or a combination of 0.5 mg ranibizumab and focal/grid laser. Group 1, 42 patients, received 0.5 mg ranibizumab at baseline and months 1, 3, and 5. Group 2, 42 patients, received focal/grid laser photocoagulation at baseline and month 3 if needed (center subfield thickness was >250 μm). Group 3, 42 patients, received a combination of 0.5 mg ranibizumab and focal/grid laser at baseline and month 3. The primary outcome was the change in BCVA at month 6 in comparison with baseline. At month 6, the group receiving ranibizumab alone showed a significant improvement in mean BCVA with respect to the patients receiving focal/grid laser. The group receiving combined therapy was not statistically different from groups 1 or 2. Resolutions of 50, 33, and 45% of excess foveal thickening were assessed in groups 1, 2, and 3, respectively. The RESOLVE study was specifically designed to evaluate the efficacy and safety of ranibizumab 0.5 mg in patients with visual impairment due to DME. The RESOLVE trial (a randomized, double-masked, multicenter, phase 2 study assessing the safety and efficacy of two concentrations of ranibizumab compared with non-treatment control for the treatment of DME with center involvement) evaluated the effect of ranibizumab on retinal edema and visual acuity (VA) in 151 patients with clinically significant DME. Patients with a central macular thickness of ≥300 μm were randomized to receive three monthly injections with either 0.3 or 0.5 mg ranibizumab or placebo. After the three monthly intravitreal injections, treatment was administrated on *pro re nata* basis for 9 months. The primary endpoint in the 1-year study was visual function at 6 months. The study design allowed the investigator to double the dose of ranibizumab if after 1 month the resolution of macular edema was incomplete. Moreover, retinal photocoagulation could be administered if needed.

The preliminary results were partially presented at the 2009 ARVO Meeting [19]. During the 12-month follow-up period, mean BCVA increased and mean CRT decreased continuously over time. The mean change in BCVA from baseline to the 12-month examination was –1.4 letters in the sham group. The groups receiving 0.3 and 0.5 mg gained, respectively, 11.8 and 8.8 letters. In order to provide further clarity on the effectiveness of treatments based on administration of steroidal or anti-VEGF drugs in comparison to conventional laser treatment, the DRCR net has designed a randomized, multicenter clinical trial which addressed the effects on visual acuity and on central retinal thickness in four groups receiving, respectively, intravitreal ranibizumab alone or associated with laser photocoagulation or triamcinolone associated with the laser treatment or laser treatment alone.

The study recruited 691 patients and examined a total of 854 eyes in a follow-up period of 2 years. Two hundred ninety-three eyes were randomized to received laser alone, 187 eyes were assigned to the group receiving 0.5 mg ranibizumab + prompt laser, 188 eyes received 0.5 mg ranibizumab + deferred laser (at least 24 weeks), and 186 eye were included in the group receiving 4 mg intravitreal triamcinolone + prompt laser.

At 1-year examination, the mean change in the visual acuity letter score respect to the baseline value showed a statistically significant improvement in the ranibizumab + prompt laser group (+9±11 letters) and ranibizumab + deferred laser group (+9±12) but not in the triamcinolone + prompt laser group (+4±13) compared with the laser group (+3±13).

Over the 2 years of follow-up a different correlation between visual acuity change and retinal thickness was observed in each group. A progressive reduction in mean central subfield thickness was noted in the laser group during the 24 months of follow-up; however, the mean change in visual acuity did not continue to increase from the 1- to 2-year visit as noted instead during the first year of follow-up.

In the triamcinolone + laser group, during the first year of follow-up an improvement of visual function was associated with a significant reduction in CST whereas from the 1- to 2-year examination the mean CST increased in parallel with a visual acuity reduction.

Ranibizumab groups showed a parallel visual acuity improvement associated with a CST reduction from baseline to 12-month visit and following the OCT results remained relatively stable up to 24-month examination and paralleled the visual acuity outcomes during this time.

Intraocular hypertension and cataract surgery were more frequently noted in the triamcinolone + prompt laser group in comparison to groups receiving ranibizumab + laser or laser alone.

The current large prospective randomized clinical trial confirms the preliminary promising results in the treatment of DME and suggests as a combined therapy might offer a more efficacious approach in this disorder where the multi-factorial pathogenesis involves several processes [20].

Actually, several multicenter international clinical trials (e.g. RESTORE, RIDE and RISE) are ongoing in order to evaluate the efficacy and safety of ranibizumab 0.5 mg as monotherapy or in combination with laser photocoagulation in eyes affected by DME.

With regard to the effects of ranibizumab on proliferative diabetic retinopathy (PDR), no studies are available in the literature evaluating this topic. However, DRCR.net has designed a prospective, randomized, comparative clinical trial to evaluate the role of ranibizumab or triamcinolone intravitreal injection as adjunctive treatment to panretinal photocoagulation for PDR.

Pegaptanib

Pegaptanib is a pegylated 28-nucleotide RNA aptamer that binds to the $VEGF_{164/165}$ isoform at high affinity. $VEGF_{165}$ levels are present in human eyes affected by DR with increased concentration and play an active role in promoting angiogenesis and in enhancing vascular permeability. Initially, pegaptanib was employed only in the treatment of neovascular age macular degeneration, where it obtained the approval of the Food and Drug Administration. Considering the role of $VEGF_{165}$ in DR and the safety and tolerability profile of intravitreally administered pegaptanib, a phase II trial was specifically designed to investigate the effects of pegaptanib in the management of DME.

The Macugen Diabetic Retinopathy Study was a randomized, sham-controlled, double-masked, dose-finding phase II trial designed to evaluate the effect of three doses of intravitreal pegaptanib vs. sham injection in patients affected by clinically significant DME [21]. The patients were randomized to receive 0.3, 1.0 or 3.0 mg of pegaptanib or sham injection at baseline, week 6 or week 12. If needed, further injections were administrated every 6 weeks up to a maximum of three additional injections. Retinal laser photocoagulation could be delivered if the investigators judged it to be necessary. The main outcome measures were changes in BCVA, central retinal thickness as assessed by OCT measurement, and additional therapy with photocoagulation between weeks 12 and 36. At the final visit at week 36, the group of patients receiving pegaptanib 0.3 mg was significantly superior to sham injection, as measured by mean change in VA (+4.7 vs. –0.4 letters; p = 0.04), proportions of patients gaining >10 letters of VA (34 vs. 10%; p = 0.003), change in mean central retinal thickness (68 μm reduction vs. 3.7 μm increase; p = 0.02). Moreover, only 25% of patients receiving pegaptanib required retinal photocoagulation in comparison with 40% of patients receiving a sham injection (p = 0.04). It is noteworthy that patients receiving 1.0 or 3.0 mg did not show a significant improvement compared to 0.3 mg with regard to BCVA or CRT changes. In general, pegaptanib was well tolerated at various concentrations; endophthalmitis occurred in 1 of 652 injections and was successfully treated without severe visual loss.

The Macugen Diabetic Retinopathy Study also provided new information on the ability of pegaptanib sodium to lead to regression of retinal neovascularization in proliferative DR [22]. Of 16 patients having retinal neovascularization in the study eye at baseline, 13 were assigned to receive pegaptanib treatment and 3 were assigned to sham injections. At 36 weeks, 8 of 13 (62%) in the pegaptanib treatment group showed regression of neovascularization, as assessed by fundus photography or fluorescein angiography, whereas no such regression occurred in 3 sham-treated eyes. In 3 of 8 with regression, neovascularization progressed at week 52 after cessation of pegaptanib at week 30, suggesting the necessity of repeated injections to control retinal neovascularization.

More recently, Gonzalez et al. [23] reported the results of a prospective, randomized, controlled, open-label, exploratory study designed to compare the efficacy of intravitreal pegaptanib vs. panretinal laser photocoagulation (PRP) in the treatment of active PDR. 20 subjects with active PDR were assigned at a 1:1 ratio to receive pegaptanib treatment in 1 eye every 6 weeks for 30 weeks or with PRP. In 90% of eyes randomized to pegaptanib, retinal neovascularization showed a complete regression by week 3. By week 12, in all eyes receiving pegaptanib a complete regression of retinal proliferation was obtained and preserved through week 36. In the PRP-treated group, at the 9-month examination, 25% demonstrated complete regression, 25% showed partial regression, and 50% showed persistent active PDR.

With regard to BCVA and although the difference between the groups was not statistically significant (p = 0.22), pegaptanib-treated eyes showed an increase of 5.8 letters in BCVA at 36 weeks, whereas the PRP-treated eyes lost 6.0 letters.

Bevacizumab

Bevacizumab is a full-length recombinant humanized antibody active against all isoforms of VEGF and currently it is approved for the treatment of metastatic colon cancer. However, anti-VEGF treatment approved for wet AMD, ranibizumab and pegaptanib is restricted in many countries; this situation has induced many retinal specialists to off-label use of bevacizumab and contemporarily it has allowed to underline the role of this VEGF antagonist in many retinal disorders including neovascular AMD, macular edema in non-ischemic central retinal vein occlusion, pseudophakic cystoid macular edema and DR.

Short-term effects of bevacizumab for DME in a large randomized phase II clinical trial were initially reported by the Diabetic Retinopathy Clinical Research Network [24]. 109 subjects with DME and Snellen acuity equivalent ranging from 20/32 to 20/320 were prospectively enrolled and randomized to 1 of 5 groups: (a) focal photocoagulation at baseline, (b) intravitreal injection of 1.25 mg bevacizumab at baseline and 6 weeks, (c) intravitreal injection of 2.5 mg bevacizumab at baseline and 6 weeks, (d) intravitreal injection of 1.25 mg bevacizumab at baseline and sham injection at 6 weeks, or (e) intravitreal injection of 1.25 mg bevacizumab at baseline and 6 weeks with photocoagulation at 3 weeks.

BCVA in groups receiving bevacizumab alone showed a median one-line improvement at the 3-week visit, which was preserved up to 12 weeks and was greater than the change in the group receiving only focal photocoagulation at baseline. A similar trend was observed with regard to central retinal thickness; comparing focal photocoagulation vs. bevacizumab alone, a greater reduction in central retina thickness was observed in the bevacizumab groups at 3 weeks. Subsequently, only a trend towards a greater reduction at 6, 9, and 12 weeks was detected.

No significant differences among groups receiving bevacizumab 1.25 vs. 2.5 mg for changes in BCVA or central retinal thickness were observed. Moreover, no meaningful differences were found comparing bevacizumab groups with groups receiving combined treatment in reduction in central subfield thickening or improvement in VA. Also, Lam et al. [25] evaluated the efficacy of two dosing regimens of bevacizumab at the 6-month follow-up. 48 patients were randomized to receive three monthly intravitreal injections of 1.25 or 2.5 mg bevacizumab. At each monthly scheduled visit a significant mean central foveal thickness reduction was observed in both groups. Similarly, mean logMAR BCVA showed a statistically significant improvement from baseline to the final visit at 6 months (from 0.63 to 0.52 in the 1.25-mg group and from 0.60 to 0.47 in the 2.5-mg group). No significant difference in BCVA was observed between the two groups. Moreover, the study confirmed the effects of bevacizumab when the intravitreal injection reached a plateau of action at 3 weeks with a subsequent decline, and repeated injections were necessary to maintain the initial effect.

More recently, Arevalo et al. [26] reported the results of a retrospective, multicenter, interventional, comparative case series with a long-term follow-up that extended to

24 months. The study evaluated 139 eyes that underwent an intravitreal injection of 1.25 or 2.5 mg bevacizumab. The main outcome measures were central foveal thickness as measured by OCT and changes in BCVA. Additional injections were administered if recurrence of macular edema was detected on OCT associated with VA loss.

At 1 month, both groups showed a statistically significant improvement in BCVA and subsequently the gain was preserved up to the 24-month examination. The 1.25-mg group improved from 20/150 to 20/107 at 1 month, and to 20/75 at 24 months. In the 2.5-mg group, BCVA improved from 20/168 to 20/118 at 1 month, and to 20/114 at the final visit. OCT examination evidenced a good anatomical response in both groups. At 1 month, the mean central macular thickness measurements decreased significantly from 446 to 333 μm; during the subsequent period a similar trend was observed up to 24 months with a final mean value of 279.7 μm. Similar results were observed in the 2.5-mg group. Over the 24-month follow-up period, 807 injections were performed and the mean number of injections per eye was 5.8 (range 1–15) at a mean interval of 12.2 ± 10.4 weeks.

Long-term efficacy of repeated injections of intravitreal 1.25 mg bevacizumab for the treatment of chronic diffuse DME was also reported by Kook et al. [27]. The study included 126 patients affected by chronic, diffuse, clinically significant DME in part not responsive to previous treatments including laser photocoagulation (62% focal laser treatment, 38% panretinal laser treatment), triamcinolone intravitreal injection (41%) or vitrectomy (11%). 67 and 59 patients completed the scheduled visits to 6 and 12 months, respectively. At the 6-month examination, logMAR BCVA ranged from a baseline value of 0.82 to 0.74 considering all patients. The mean BCVA of patients who completed the 12-month follow-up improved similarly from 0.82 to 0.74. Mean central retinal thickness decreased from 463 to 374 μm after 6 months, and to 357 μm after 12 months with a statistically significant difference. The authors concluded that even in cases with chronic diffuse ischemic DME not responding to other therapies, a successful treatment with repeated intravitreal injections of bevacizumab can be observed in a long-term follow-up.

Other studies compared intravitreal bevacizumab treatment with intravitreal triamcinolone or focal retinal photocoagulation in refractory DME or as primary treatment. Paccola et al. [28] designed a randomized, prospective study in order to evaluate the anatomical response and VA outcomes after a single intravitreal injection of 4 mg triamcinolone acetonide or 1.25 mg bevacizumab in the refractory diffuse DME. The study enrolled 26 patients; at baseline, logMAR BCVA was 0.936 and 0.937 in the triamcinolone and bevacizumab groups, respectively. At 6 months, BCVA improved to 0.91 and 0.92 without achieving a significant difference; however, interim analysis at the 1-, 2- and 3-month examinations evidenced a significant improvement in the triamcinolone group in comparison with the bevacizumab group. Central macular thickness was significantly reduced in the intravitreal triamcinolone group compared with the bevacizumab group at weeks 4, 8, 12 and 24. The analysis of changes in CMT over the follow-up showed a significant from baseline at weeks 4, 8 and 12 in the triamcinolone group and at weeks 4 and 8 in the bevacizumab group.

A similar prospective and comparative case series was reported by Shimura et al. [29]. The study recruited 14 patients with bilateral long-standing DME; in each patient, 1 eye was selected to receive a single intravitreal injection of triamcinolone (4 mg) and the other to receive a single intravitreal bevacizumab injection (1.25 mg).

logMAR BCVA in the triamcinolone group improved significantly from 0.64 to 0.33 at 1 week, and the gain was subsequently preserved up to 12 weeks. At a final observation period of 24 weeks, BCVA decreased to 0.47 but was still significantly different from the baseline value. Similarly, BCVA in the bevacizumab group improved from 0.61 to 0.39 at 1 week and maintained the initial gain up to 4 weeks. At 12 weeks, BCVA returned to the initial level. No further decrease or improvement was observed in the following 3 months. Between the two groups, a statistically significant difference of BCVA was observed in favor of the triamcinolone group at 3 and 6 months.

Morphological analysis revealed a significant decrease of foveal thickness from 522 to 342.6 μm in the triamcinolone group at 1 week. At 12 weeks the foveal thickness maintained the improvement, but at 6 months it increased slightly to 410.4 μm. The bevacizumab group showed a significant foveal thickness reduction at 1 week from 527 to 397 μm and preserved the improvement also at 4 weeks. In the following weeks, the foveal thickness showed a progressive worsening and reached the initial level at 12 weeks; no further worsening or improvement was observed in the following 12 weeks. Between the two groups, a statistically significant difference of foveal thickness was observed in favor of the triamcinolone group at 1, 3 and 6 months.

A more recently, randomized, three-arm clinical trial comparing intravitreal bevacizumab injection (1.25 mg) alone or in combination with intravitreal triamcinolone acetonide (2 mg) versus macular laser photocoagulation as a primary treatment of DME was published by Soheilian et al. [30]. Each arm enrolled 50 patients receiving the treatment at baseline and at 12 weeks as needed. The main outcome measure was change in BCVA at the 4-month examination, but the study also provided the results at 36 weeks. The bevacizumab group showed a significant BCVA improvement from 0.71 to 0.54 at 6 weeks; the initial gain was maintained at each following visit at 12, 24 and 36 weeks. The patients who underwent to combined treatment showed a significant BCVA improvement from 0.73 to 0.60 at 6 weeks. This group maintained BCVA also at 12 weeks but lost the statistically significant improvement at 6 and 9 months. In the macular photocoagulation group, BCVA showed a stabilization at 6 weeks in comparison to the baseline value (0.60 vs. 0.55) and similar values were observed at all follow-up visits; however, we should consider that the three groups differed with regard to the baseline VA values.

The mean values of central macular thickness decreased significantly in all groups only at 6 weeks in comparison to the baseline values and although the reduction was greater in the bevacizumab group with respect to the other two groups, no statistically significant differences were registered at any of the follow-ups among the three groups. Retreatment was administered to 27 eyes up to 6 months and specifically 14 eyes received an additional bevacizumab injection, 10 eyes received combined treatment and macular photocoagulation was performed in 3 eyes.

Another interesting element of this study is represented by regression of retinal neovascularization that presented initially in 9 patients. After the first bevacizumab treatment, the neovascularization resolved in all subjects. Treatment of retinal neovascularization associated with DR has been the object of study in several investigations exploring the employment of bevacizumab as an antiangiogenic drug.

In a retrospective study, Avery et al. [31] investigated the biologic effects of intravitreal bevacizumab in patients with retinal and iris neovascularization secondary to diabetes mellitus in 45 eyes. The patients received intravitreal bevacizumab in a dose-escalating regimen (6.2 g to 1.25 mg). Changes in fluorescein angiographic leakage and in BCVA were the primary and secondary outcome, respectively. At the 1-week examination, fluorescein angiography disclosed a complete or at least partial reduction in leakage of the neovascularization. Recurrence was registered in variable time: in 1 case recurrence of retinal neovascularization was detected after 2 weeks whereas in the other cases no recurrent leakage was registered at the last follow-up of 11 weeks.

In a prospective, non-randomized open-label study, Jorge et al. [32] evaluated the effects of bevacizumab in patients affected by active proliferative DR refractory to laser treatment and with a BCVA value inferior to 20/40. Each patient received a single intravitreal bevacizumab injection of 1.5 mg. 15 patients completed the scheduled visits up to 12 weeks of follow-up. Mean logMAR BCVA improved significantly from 0.90 at baseline to 0.76 at week 1; subsequently the improvement was preserved up to the 12-week examination. At baseline the mean neovascularization leakage area was 27.79 mm^2. At the 1- and 12-week examinations, the mean neovascularization leakage area decreased significantly to 5.43 and 5.50, respectively.

Additional data on the use of bevacizumab in patients affected by proliferative DR complicated by vitreous hemorrhages has been provided by Moradian et al. [33]. 38 patients were enrolled and prospectively followed up to 20 weeks. Mean logMAR BCVA increased from 1.13 to 0.86 1 week after the injection; a further improvement was observed at 6, 12 and 20 weeks, with a final mean value of 0.53. Vitreous hemorrhages resolved significantly at the 1- and 12-week examinations and about 50% of patients showed a complete resolution. At 20 weeks, only the 23% of the eyes presented a slight degree of vitreous hemorrhages.

A more recent investigation corroborates these results. Huang et al. [34] evaluated the efficacy of intravitreal bevacizumab combined with panretinal photocoagulation in the treatment of PDR complicated by vitreous hemorrhage. In their prospective study, 40 patients underwent an intravitreal bevacizumab injection (1.25 mg) followed by PRP. An additional injection was administered if no signs of decreased vitreous hemorrhages were noted. In the event of persistent vitreous hemorrhage over 12 weeks, vitrectomy was performed. The vitreous clear-up time and rate of vitrectomy were registered and compared with the control group treated with conventional methods. The vitreous clear-up time in the bevacizumab group was significantly lower than in the control group (11.9 vs. 18.1 weeks). Similarly, the bevacizumab group required vitrectomy in 10% of the patients compared to 45% of the control group. 31 and 9 patients respectively received 1 and 2 injections.

VEGF Trap

The VEGF Trap-Eye (Regeneron Inc.) is a 115-kDa recombinant fusion protein of portions of VEGF receptors 1 and 2, and the Fc region of human IgG which binds all VEGF-A isoforms with higher affinity in comparison to other anti-VEGFs, including bevacizumab and ranibizumab [35]. Moreover, VEGF Trap-Eye has a longer half-life in the eye after intraocular injection and it binds other members of the VEGF family including placental growth factors 1 and 2, which have been shown to contribute to excessive vascular permeability. This higher affinity will probably allow to employ lower doses and to maintain a longer duration of action [36, 37].

A study phase I exploring the safety and bioactivity of a single injection of 4.0 mg VEGF Trap-Eye in subjects with DME has been reported by Do et al. [38]. At 4 weeks, 5 of the 5 subjects showed a good anatomical response with a meaningful reduction in excess retinal foveal thickness. All but 1 subject maintained the reduction at 6 weeks after the injection. The median improvement in BCVA was 9 letters on the ETDRS chart at 1 month and 3 letters at 6 weeks. In general, a single intravitreal injection of 4.0 mg VEGF Trap-Eye was well tolerated and no serious ocular adverse events were reported. An extended phase II study on a larger sample of patients and with a longer follow-up is waited with great interest.

Bevasiranib

Small interfering RNA (siRNA) molecules are able to inactive the RNA messenger and suppress RNA translation. Bevasiranib is a specific siRNA designed to decrease the level and activity of VEGF mRNA. In this regard, bevasiranib may have a role in the treatment of DR [39–41].

The RACE trial was a double-masked, randomized, phase 2 study, designed to investigate the safety and efficacy of bevasiranib in patients with DME [42]. At the end of the follow-up, 48 patients had completed the scheduled visit. Each patient was assigned to one of three arms receiving respectively bevasiranib 0.2, 1.5 or 3.0 mg. Bevasiranib was administered monthly for 3 months. Primary and secondary outcome measures were changes on macular edema as measured by OCT and on BCVA. In this pilot study, there was a trend showing a decrease in macular thickness between weeks 8 and 12, where the higher doses result in a larger reduction in thickness than the lowest dose. BCVA showed a stabilization in 91% of patients. No severe side effect was observed, however 4 patients reported mild uveitis.

Rapamycin

Rapamycin is a macrocyclic antibiotic produced by the bacterium *Streptomyces hygroscopicus* and found in the soil of Easter Island and it was initially classified as a macrolide fungicide; nevertheless, it shows a wide range of actions including immunosuppressive, antitumor and antiangiogenic properties. Rapamycin binds specifically the FKBP12; the active complex inhibits the mammalian target of rapamycin (mTOR), a kinase, which integrates growth factor-activated signals including signals promoting angiogenesis mediated by VEGF. Moreover, mTOR is an activator of hypoxia-inducible factor 1a, which upregulates the transcription of VEGF. In hypoxic cells, rapamycin can interfere with HIF-1a activation by increasing the rate of its degradation [43–45].

In essence, the antiangiogenic properties of rapamycin are associated with a decrease in VEGF production and a reduction in the response of vascular endothelial cells to stimulation by VEGF. Rapamycin may therefore have a meaningful role as therapy for retinal disorders characterized by pathological vascular permeability and proliferation. Preliminary results of application of rapamycin for DME were presented at the 2008 ARVO Meeting by Blumenkranz et al. [46]. A multicenter, open-label phase 1 dose-escalation study was designed with the aim of evaluating the safety and pharmacological activity of rapamycin. 50 patients were randomly assigned to receive either a single intravitreal (44, 110, 176, 264, or 352 μg) or a single subconjunctival (220, 440, 880, 1,320, or 1,760 μg) rapamycin injection. The primary outcome was changes in BCVA evaluated on the ETDRS chart and changes on central retinal thickness evaluated by OCT at 14, 45, 90 and 180 days. With regard to BCVA, a significant improvement was observed at 14, 45 and 90 days in both groups receiving a 440-μg subconjunctival injection and the group receiving a 352-μg intravitreal injection. Specifically, the intravitreal injection group showed a mean gain of 11.6, 6.4, and 7.8 letters at 14, 45 and 90 days. The subconjunctival injection group gained 8.8, 11.4, and 7.4 letters. A significant central macular thickness reduction was observed in both groups with mean OCT reductions of 33, 78, and 54 μm in the patients receiving a subconjunctival injection and 72, 42, and 61 μm in the patients receiving an intravitreal injection. No dose-limiting toxicities were observed and no serious ocular adverse events were registered.

Conclusion

Anti-VEGF therapy has opened a new perspective in the treatment of DME and of proliferative retinopathy. However, the pathogenesis and the course of the DR will demand a more complex approach. Currently, retinal laser photocoagulation is the only recommended treatment in the clinically significant macular edema and in PDR. These statements are derived from large clinical randomized, controlled trials which are not available for the pharmacological classes analyzed above [47]. For each molecule, anti-VEGF must be defined as the more effective scheme of administration in reference to the characteristics of the single molecules, the dosing, and for some also the routes of administration; moreover, the use of selective vs. non-selective molecules has to be better defined. A better definition of anti-VEGF treatment in reference to the characteristics and stadiation of DR is necessary; thus, more specific inclusion and exclusion criteria are required including the presence of early or advanced DR, duration of symptoms and signs, visual function, presence of concomitant retinal edema and proliferation, and previous treatments. A head-to-head comparison between anti-VEGF and conventional laser therapy is necessary, and, considering the multifactor pathogenesis, verification of the effectiveness of combined treatments, including laser treatment and corticosteroid therapy, is needed.

Finally, the surgical approach could receive additional support in the management of complications of advanced DR, neovascular glaucoma and in the progression of macular edema associated with cataract surgery.

References

1 Kempen JH, O'Colmain BJ, Leske MC, et al: Eye Diseases Prevalence Research Group: The prevalence of diabetic retinopathy among adults in the United States. Arch Ophthalmol 2004;122:552–563.

2 Klein R: Retinopathy in a population-based study. Trans Am Ophthalmol Soc 1992;90:561–594.

3 Orchard TJ, Dorman JS, Maser RE, et al: Prevalence of complications in IDDM by sex and duration. Pittsburgh Epidemiology of Diabetes Complications Study II. Diabetes 1990;39:1116–1124.

4 Wild S, Roglic G, Green A, Sicree R, et al: Global prevalence of diabetes: estimates for the year 2000 and projections for 2030. Diabetes Care 2004;27: 1047–1053.

5 Caldwell RB, Bartoli M, Behzadian MA, et al: Vascular endothelial growth factor and diabetic retinopathy: pathophysiological mechanisms and treatment perspectives. Diabetes Metab Res Rev 2003;19:442–455.

6 Lu M, Kuroki M, Amano S, et al: Advanced glycation end products increase retinal vascular endothelial growth factor expression. J Clin Invest 1998;101: 1219–1224.

7 Gabbay KH: The sorbitol pathway and the complications of diabetes. N Engl J Med 1973;288:831–836.

8 Gardner TW, Antonetti DA, Barber AJ, et al: Diabetic retinopathy: more than meets the eye. Surv Ophthalmol 2002;47(suppl 2):253–262.

9 Aiello LP, Northrup JM, Keyt BA, et al: Hypoxic regulation of vascular endothelial growth factor in retinal cells. Arch Ophthalmol 1995;113:1538–1544.

10 Neufeld G, Cohen T, Gengrinovitch S, et al: Vascular endothelial growth factor and its receptors. FASEB J 1999,13:9–22.

11 Grant MB, Afzal A, Spoerri P, et al: The role of growth factors in the pathogenesis of diabetic retinopathy. Expert Opin Investig Drugs 2004;13:1275–1293.

12 Plate KH, Breier G, Weich HA, et al: Vascular endothelial growth factor is a potential tumour angiogenesis factor in human gliomas in vivo. Nature 1992 29;359:845–848.

13 Shweiki D, Itin A, Soffer D, et al: Vascular endothelial growth factor induced by hypoxia may mediate hypoxia-initiated angiogenesis. Nature 1992;359: 843–845.

14 Aiello LP, Avery RL, Arrigg PG, et al: Vascular endothelial growth factor in ocular fluid of patients with diabetic retinopathy and other retinal disorders. N Engl J Med 1994;331:1480–1487.

15 Ferrara N: Vascular endothelial growth factor: basic science and clinical progress. Endocr Rev 2004;25: 581–611.

16 Chun DW, Heier JS, Topping TM, et al: A pilot study of multiple intravitreal injections of ranibizumab in patients with center-involving clinically significant diabetic macular edema. Ophthalmology 2006;113: 1706–1712.

17 Nguyen QD, Tatlipinar S, Shah SM, et al: Vascular endothelial growth factor is a critical stimulus for diabetic macular edema. Am J Ophthalmol 2006; 142:961–969.

18 Nguyen QD, Shah SM, Heier JS, et al: READ-2 Study Group: Primary endpoint (6 months) results of the ranibizumab for edema of the macula in diabetes (READ-2) study. Ophthalmology 2009;116: 2175–21781.e1.

19 Wolf A, Massin P, Bandello F, et al: RESOLVE Study Group: Safety and efficacy of ranibizumab treatment in patients with diabetic macular edema: 12-month results of the RESOLVE study. ARVO Meeting, Fort Lauderdale, 2009.
20 The Diabetic Retinopathy Clinical Research Network, Elman MJ, Aiello LP, Beck RW, Bressler NM, Bressler SB, Edwards AR, Ferris FL 3rd, Friedman SM, Glassman AR, Miller KM, Scott IU, Stockdale CR, Sun JK: Randomized Trial Evaluating Ranibizumab Plus Prompt or Deferred Laser or Triamcinolone Plus Prompt Laser for Diabetic Macular Edema. Ophthalmology 2010;117:1064 –1077.
21 Cunningham ET Jr, Adamis AP, Altaweel M, et al: Macugen Diabetic Retinopathy Study Group: A phase II randomized double-masked trial of pegaptanib, an antivascular endothelial growth factor aptamer, for diabetic macular edema. Ophthalmology 2005;112:1747–1757.
22 Adamis AP, Altaweel M, Bressler NM, et al: Macugen Diabetic Retinopathy Study Group: Changes in retinal neovascularization after pegaptanib (Macugen) therapy in diabetic individuals. Ophthalmology 2006;113:23–28.
23 Gonzalez VH, Giuliari GP, Banda RM, et al: Intravitreal injection of pegaptanib sodium for proliferative diabetic retinopathy. Br J Ophthalmol 2009;93:1474–1478.
24 Diabetic Retinopathy Clinical Research Network: A phase II randomized clinical trial of intravitreal bevacizumab for diabetic macular edema. Ophthalmology 2007;114:1860–1867.
25 Lam DS, Lai TY, Lee VY, et al: Efficacy of 1.25 vs. 2.5 mg intravitreal bevacizumab for diabetic macular edema: six-month results of a randomized controlled trial. Retina 2009;29:292–299.
26 Arevalo JF, Sanchez JG, Wu L, et al: Pan-American Collaborative Retina Study Group: Primary intravitreal bevacizumab for diffuse diabetic macular edema: the Pan-American Collaborative Retina Study Group at 24 months. Ophthalmology 2009; 116:1488–1497.
27 Kook D, Wolf A, Kreutzer T, et al: Long-term effect of intravitreal bevacizumab (Avastin) in patients with chronic diffuse diabetic macular edema. Retina 2008;28:1053–1060.
28 Paccola L, Costa RA, Folgosa MS, et al: Intravitreal triamcinolone versus bevacizumab for treatment of refractory diabetic macular oedema (IBEME study). Br J Ophthalmol 2008;92:76–80.
29 Shimura M, Nakazawa T, Yasuda K, et al: Comparative therapy evaluation of intravitreal bevacizumab and triamcinolone acetonide on persistent diffuse diabetic macular edema. Am J Ophthalmol 2008;145:854–861.
30 Soheilian M, Ramezani A, Obudi A, et al: Randomized trial of intravitreal bevacizumab alone or combined with triamcinolone versus macular photocoagulation in diabetic macular edema. Ophthalmology 2009;116:1142–1150.
31 Avery RL, Pearlman J, Pieramici DJ, et al: Intravitreal bevacizumab (Avastin) in the treatment of proliferative diabetic retinopathy. Ophthalmology 2006;113: 1695.e1–15.
32 Jorge R, Costa RA, Calucci D, et al: Intravitreal bevacizumab (Avastin) for persistent new vessels in diabetic retinopathy (IBEPE study). Retina 2006;26: 1006–1013.
33 Moradian S, Ahmadieh H, Malihi M, et al: Intravitreal bevacizumab in active progressive proliferative diabetic retinopathy. Graefes Arch Clin Exp Ophthalmol 2008;246:1699–1705.
34 Huang YH, Yeh PT, Chen MS, et al: Intravitreal bevacizumab and panretinal photocoagulation for proliferative diabetic retinopathy associated with vitreous haemorrhage. Retina 2009;29:1134–1140.
35 Economides AN, Carpenter LR, Rudge JS, et al: Cytokine traps: multi-component, high-affinity blockers of cytokine action. Nat Med 2003;9:47–52.
36 Holash J, Davis S, Papadopoulos N, et al: VEGF Trap: a VEGF blocker with potent antitumor effects. Proc Natl Acad Sci USA 2002;99:11393–11398.
37 Stewart MW, Rosenfeld PJ: Predicted biological activity of intravitreal VEGF Trap. Br J Ophthalmol 2008;92:667–668.
38 Do DV, Nguyen QD, Shah SM, et al: An exploratory study of the safety, tolerability and bioactivity of a single intravitreal injection of vascular endothelial growth factor Trap-eye in patients with diabetic macular oedema. Br J Ophthalmol 2009;93:144–149.
39 Reich SJ, Fosnot J, Kuroki A, et al: Small interfering RNA targeting VEGF effectively inhibits ocular neovascularization in a mouse model. Mol Vis 2003; 9:210–216.
40 Shen J, Samul R, Silva RL, et al: Suppression of ocular neovascularization with siRNA targeting VEGF receptor 1. Gene Ther 2006;13:225–234.
41 Singerman LJ: Combination therapy using the small interfering RNA bevasiranib. Retina 2009;29(suppl): 49–50.
42 Singerman LJ: Intravitreal bevasiranib in exudative age-related macular degeneration or diabetic macular edema. 25th Annual Meeting of the American Society of Retina Specialists, Indian Wells, December 1–5, 2007.
43 Sausville EA, Elsayed Y, Monga M, et al: Signal transduction-directed cancer treatments. Annu Rev Pharmacol Toxicol 2003;43:199–231.

44 Guba M, von Breitenbuch P, Steinbauer M, et al: Rapamycin inhibits primary and metastatic tumor growth by antiangiogenesis: involvement of vascular endothelial growth factor. Nat Med 2002;8:128–135.
45 Sehgal SN: Rapamune (RAPA, rapamycin, sirolimus): mechanism of action immunosuppressive effect results from blockade of signal transduction and inhibition of cell cycle progression. Clin Biochem 1998;31:335–340.
46 Blumenkranz MS, Dugel PU, Solley WA, et al: A randomized dose-escalation trial of locally-administered sirolimus to treat diabetic macular edema. 2008 Annual Meeting of the Association of Research in Vision and Ophthalmology, Fort Lauderdale 2008, v49.
47 Early Treatment Diabetic Retinopathy Study (ETDRS) Research Group: Treatment techniques and clinical guidelines for photocoagulation of diabetic macular edema. ETDRS Report No. 2. Ophthalmology 1987;94:761–774.

Francesco Bandello, MD, FEBO
Professor and Chairman, Department of Ophthalmology
University Vita-Salute Scientific Institute, San Raffaele
Via Olgettina, 60, IT–20132 Milan (Italy)
Tel. +39 02 2643 2648, Fax +39 02 2648 3643, E-Mail francesco.bandello@hsr.it

Bandello F, Battaglia Parodi M (eds): Anti-VEGF.
Dev Ophthalmol. Basel, Karger, 2010, vol 46, pp 54–72

Retinal Vein Occlusions

Wolf Buehl · Stefan Sacu · Ursula Schmidt-Erfurth

Department of Ophthalmology and Optometry, Medical University Vienna,
Vienna, Austria

Abstract

Retinal vein occlusion (RVO) is a common cause of vision loss in elderly people. The complex pathogenesis of central RVO (CRVO), hemi-RVO (HRVO) and branch RVO (BRVO) makes it an interdisciplinary task. Treatment of RVO should aim at eliminating the complications and vision-disturbing effects of RVO but also include prophylactic measures in order to avoid recurrence of the disease. Problems are mainly caused by the ischemic form of RVO, leading to neovascularization. Several treatment methods have been investigated over the past decades, including drug therapy and surgical methods. Until recently, sufficient evidence-based studies were only available for the effect of grid and scatter laser therapy on RVO. New studies have shown a positive effect of intravitreal therapy with vascular endothelial growth factor inhibitors (anti-VEGF therapy) on the progression of the disease. Ongoing studies are now focusing on different combination therapies. Larger randomized studies will hopefully lead to a commonly accepted regimen for treatment of CRVO and BRVO in the near future.

Background

Retinal vein occlusion (RVO) is the second most common vascular retinal disease, following diabetic retinopathy [1, 2]. There are three types of RVO: central RVO (CRVO), hemi-RVO (HRVO), and branch RVO (BRVO). The prevalence of CRVO ranges from 0.1 to 0.4 in the population aged 40 and older. BRVO occurs three times more often than CRVO and is a common reason for (unilateral) decreased visual acuity in elderly people [3, 4]. The average age at the first occurrence lies around 70 years. Patients suffer from reduced visual acuity and visual field defects. The decrease in visual acuity is caused by macular edema, macular ischemia, vitreous hemorrhage, retinal hemorrhages, development of epiretinal membranes, or retinal degeneration [1]. Complications of RVO include vitreous hemorrhage, rubeosis iridis and neovascularization glaucoma.

RVO leads to reduced or missing outflow of venous blood, followed by retinal vascular leakage and macular edema due to an increased intracapillary pressure.

Exudation of blood components causes segmental intraretinal hemorrhages. Two occlusion types (ischemic and non-ischemic) can be distinguished [3–6]. The prevalence of BRVO lies between 0.6 and 1.6%, the incidence around 2.14 per 1,000 people aged 40 or older [3, 7–9]. The highest risk exists at the age of 60–70 years. There are no gender-specific differences [10].

The precise etiology of RVO is not entirely clear. There are five pathogenetic mechanisms which may lead to less perfusion of the retinal vein: neurovascular compression, alteration of the vascular wall, increased blood viscosity, hematologic abnormalities, and inflammation.

BRVO typically occurs at arteriovenous crossings, often being located in the superotemporal quadrant [11–13]. The main risk factors for the development of BRVO are arteriosclerotic, hypertensive and diabetic changes in retinal arterioles [6, 14]. In contrast to CRVO, local factors such as glaucoma or ocular hypertension do not seem to play an essential role in the pathogenesis of BRVO.

Although several methods of treatment have been described for RVO, most of these options lack a sufficient amount of prospective and randomized studies assessing their effectiveness and several studies do not differentiate between CRVO, HRVO and BRVO. However, there are substantial differences between CRVO and BRVO concerning visual prognosis, risk of complications and efficiency of different therapies. Laser photocoagulation has been the only evidence-based treatment for patients with macular edema secondary to BRVO and CRVO since 1984 [1, 2]. Recently, several studies focusing on the effect of intravitreal antivascular endothelial growth factor (anti-VEGF) treatment have been published.

Pathogenesis and Risk Factors

Although RVO is a common retinal vascular disorder, its precise pathogenesis is still not entirely understood. Undoubtedly, acute RVO is associated with thrombotic changes in the vascular system, leading to intraluminal narrowing and venous congestion with increased venous pressure [15]. This intravascular alteration consecutively causes a breakdown of the blood retina barrier with extravasation and typical, flame-shaped intraretinal bleedings. The barrier defect results from a primarily unobstructed arterial blood flow and simultaneously reduced venous outflow. In case of CRVO or BRVO with affection of the central retina, stasis with hypertension also causes the typical extracellular macular edema: local ischemia with expression of VEGF and related cytokines and the particular anatomic structure of the macular retina play an important role in its genesis. Depending on the severity of the vascular obstruction with concomitant capillary dropout and arteriolar alteration, retinal ischemia may develop and can lead to neovascularization.

Similar to other vascular diseases, there are three main mechanisms in the development of RVO: (degenerative) changes of the vascular wall, pathologic hematologic factors, and reduced vascular flow rate. CRVO may also be caused by neurovascular compression (increased intraocular pressure) and by inflammatory processes.

Degenerative Changes of the Vessel Wall

Histological observations revealed typical alterations of the vascular endothelium and intima media in the vicinity of arteriovenous crossings. These changes, perhaps resulting from the compression of the vein by the overlying artery, and subsequent formation of a thrombus, seem to be important steps in the genesis of RVO. Sclerosis of the retinal artery, which is often associated with systemic diseases such as hypertension, atherosclerosis, diabetes, and enhanced by smoking, may lead to further compression of the vein, resulting in turbulent blood flow causing further damage of the venous vessel wall and finally leading to formation of a thrombus. Consequently, there is a positive feedback loop between the pathogenesis of reduced vascular flow rate and that of degenerative changes of the vessel wall.

Hematologic Factors

Severe disorders of the blood components such as an increased cell count or unbalanced plasma protein levels (leukemia, polycythemia, etc.) as well as minor changes in blood viscosity – especially hyperviscosity due to increased hematocrit values (hyperviscosity syndrome) – may contribute to the pathogenesis of RVO. On the other hand, the influence of blood coagulation factors (including resistance to activated protein C and deficiency of protein C, protein S, antithrombin, and others) on the development of RVO has been discussed controversially [16–19]. Studies in elderly patients (>45 years) with blood coagulation disorders did not find a higher risk for RVO compared to a control group. However, particularly young patients (<45 years) with RVO without arteriosclerotic risk factors should be referred to a hematologist. In particular, these patients should be screened for homocysteinemia (relative risk: 8.9) and for antiphospholipid antibodies (mainly anticardiolipin antibodies) and lupus anticoagulants (relative risk: 3.9). However, in the vast majority of patients with RVO, blood and plasma parameters are unremarkable.

Reduced Vascular Flow Rate

The retinal vascular flow rate is influenced by the anatomic characteristics of the vascular architecture of the retina and at the optic nerve head. Artery and vein are located in close vicinity, sharing a common adventitia, and enter the globe through the lamina cribrosa. Therefore, sclerotic changes in the arterial wall may impede the blood flow of the adjacent vein, separating the pathogenesis of RVOs from that of peripheral vein occlusions such as deep venous thrombosis. Furthermore, it is also generally accepted that the mechanical narrowing of the venous lumen at arteriovenous crossings plays an important role in the pathogenesis of BRVO. At the majority of arteriovenous crossings, the retinal vein is located between the more rigid artery and the cellular retina.

Neurovascular Compression

Open angle glaucoma, ischemic optic neuropathy, pseudotumor cerebri, tilted optic nerve heads, and optic nerve head drusen are risk factors for the development of CRVO. Contrary to CRVO, these local risk factors do not seem to play a major role in the pathogenesis of BRVO.

Inflammation

Inflammatory/autoimmune vasculitis (systemic lupus erythematodes) as well as infectious vasculitis (sarcoidosis, HIV, syphilis, herpes zoster) may play a role in the pathogenesis of RVO. There are also a number of purely retinal causes of BRVO, namely Von Hippel's disease, Coats' disease, Eales' disease, Behçet's syndrome and toxoplasmosis. Further risk factors, which may be associated with a higher incidence of RVO, include retrobulbar block, dehydration, pregnancy, and different medications, e.g. oral contraceptives, diuretics, hepatitis B vaccine.

There are also some factors which seem to decrease the risk for RVO, including frequent physical activity, moderate alcohol consumption, higher serum levels of high-density lipoprotein cholesterol, and exogenous estrogens (in women). Table 1 summarizes the major commonly accepted risk factors for RVO. Although there is no evidence for a causal association with specific systemic diseases [20], patients should always be referred to a specialist for internal medicine to detect and treat any underlying disease and to assess the patient's risk profile with special regard to arterial hypertension and blood coagulation disorders.

Symptoms and Natural Course

Central Retinal Vein Occlusion (CRVO)

There are two types of CRVO:

(1) *Non-ischemic (perfused) CRVO (NICRVO) or venous stasis retinopathy.* Compared with eyes that have the ischemic type, eyes with NICRVO typically have a visual acuity of 20/200 or better, relatively few cotton-wool spots, and less marked retinal hemorrhage. Approximately 20% of NICRVO will progress to ischemic CRVOs. The ophthalmoscopic features are similar to ischemic CRVO, but are much less extensive. Engorgement of the venous tree (including the capillaries) is prominent; increased tortuosity and dilation of the veins and a darker appearance of the blood column are common findings; retinal hemorrhages vary markedly. Cotton-wool spots are rare. Vision may be decreased because of macular edema or macular hemorrhage.

(2) *Ischemic (non-perfused) CRVO (ICRVO) or hemorrhagic retinopathy.* ICRVO is defined by more than 9 disc areas in diameter of retinal capillary non-perfusion on angiography. 35% of ischemic eyes develop iris neovascularization or angular neovascularization. Confluent hemorrhages are concentrated in the posterior pole, many

Table 1. Supposed risk factors for RVO

Supposed risk factors for RVO
Cardiovascular diseases
Arterial hypertension
Hyperlipidemia
Diabetes mellitus
Coronary heart disease
Blood coagulation disorders
Hyperhomocysteinemia
Antiphospholipid syndrome
Resistance to activated protein C (factor V Leiden mutation)
Deficiency of antithrombin III
Mutation in the prothrombin gene (factor II)
Rheological disorders
Elevated hematocrit levels
Increased blood viscosity
Increased erythrocyte aggregation
Reduced deformability of erythrocytes
Hyperviscosity syndrome
Polycythemia vera
Waldenström macroglobulinemia
Myeloma
Leukemia
Further risk factors
Obesity
Smoking
Oral contraceptives
Glaucoma (CRVO)
Severe retinopathy (BRVO)
Abnormalities and ischemia of the optic nerve (head)
Pseudotumor cerebri
Inflammatory diseases (vasculitis)

hemorrhages are flame-shaped, and dot and punctate hemorrhages are interspersed and indicate involvement of the deeper retinal layers. Bleedings may be extensive, erupting through the internal limiting membrane to form a preretinal hemorrhage or extending into the vitreous. Typically, the entire venous tree is tortuous, engorged, dilated, and dark. The retina appears edematous, particularly in the posterior pole, and cotton-wool patches (soft exudates) are often present.

Hemicentral Vein Occlusion (HRVO)

In approximately 20% of eyes, the branch retinal veins draining the superior and inferior halves of the retina enter the lamina cribrosa separately before joining to form a single central retinal vein. HRVO is an occlusion of one of these dual trunks of the central retinal vein within the nerve. HRVO therefore involves the venous drainage from approximately half of the retina, either the superior or the inferior retina. Three factors that were significantly associated with this type of occlusion compared to control were systemic hypertension, diabetes mellitus, and glaucoma.

Branch Retinal Vein Occlusion (BRVO)

BRVO typically occurs at the intersection of a branch retinal artery with a vein. It is generally less visually disabling than CRVO or HRVO. Most BRVOs involve veins located temporal to the optic disc; there are significantly more vein-posterior than vein-anterior crossings in the superotemporal than the inferotemporal quadrant, and vein-posterior crossings are more likely to be obstructed than vein-anterior crossings.

Based on the amount of capillary non-perfusion (ischemic index) present on the fluorescein angiogram, Magargal and co-workers classified BRVO, in a manner similar to that for CRVO, into three types: (1) hyperpermeable (non-ischemic), (2) indeterminate, and (3) ischemic. The ischemic index is the percentage of non-perfused retina based on the amount of retina that is obstructed, rather than the entire retina. Hayreh and co-workers categorized BRVO as mild, moderate, and marked, based on the degree of capillary non-perfusion seen angiographically. As in CRVO, there is a spectrum of capillary non-perfusion in BRVO, ranging from little, if any, non-perfusion to extensive or almost complete non-perfusion. It is probably most clinically useful to classify eyes as non-ischemic and ischemic because neovascularization generally occurs only in the ischemic cases. The key to the diagnosis lies in the unilateral and segmental distribution of the ophthalmoscopic findings. This distribution of findings distinguishes BRVO from other disorders involving hemorrhage, cotton-wool spots, and retinal edema. Visual field defects range from relative to absolute scotomata and peripheral depression in the involved corresponding segment. Eyes with branch retinal vein obstruction and retinal capillary non-perfusion can develop neovascularization of the retina and/or disc.

Due to the compromised function of the central retina, CRVO, HRVO and major BRVO are usually characterized by a sudden onset of clinical symptoms. Patients complain about decreased visual acuity and visual field defects. Typically, these complaints are more severe in the morning, caused by the increased venous pressure (lower head position) during sleep and symptoms may disappear entirely during the day. Floaters and metamorphopsia are further typical complaints. Weeks following the initial event, a second occlusion may lead to a further decline in visual acuity. Other than CRVO and major BRVO, peripheral BRVO may remain unnoticed until complications occur.

Typical early complications of RVO with macular involvement include macular edema, macular non-perfusion and vitreous hemorrhage. Ophthalmoscopically, cotton-wool spots and lipid deposits in the retinal nerve fiber layer as well as tortuositas and dilatation of retinal veins in the affected area are common findings [4, 21].

The natural history of eyes with CRVO, particularly in older patients presenting with reduced visual acuity, is usually poor. In the Central Retinal Vein Occlusion Study, 16% of eyes developed iris and/or angle neovascularization, a total of 34% converted to the ischemic type of the disease. After 3 years of follow-up, 58% of eyes – especially in patients who initially present with poor visual acuity – will have vision worse than 20/200 [2].

The prognosis regarding visual acuity after BRVO depends mostly on the localization of the occlusion [14]. A study by the branch vein occlusion group found a spontaneous increase in visual acuity after BRVO by two or more lines (logMAR scale) in 37%, but only in 17% a decrease of 2 or more lines [1]. Subsequently, a mean increase in visual acuity of 2.3 lines was documented after 3 years. 34% of patients attained a final visual acuity of 20/40 or better, only 23% a final visual acuity below 20/200. Reasons for a recovery of visual acuity are resolution of intraretinal bleedings and cotton-wool spots, the development of collateral vessels and capillary compensation, leading to restored blood flow and resorption of retinal edema [14, 16]. The severity of the occlusion and extent of ischemia are important prognostic factors for the natural course of visual acuity after RVO [14].

Differentiation between ischemic and non-ischemic RVO is not always easy and usually cannot be made by ophthalmoscopy alone. In addition, slit-lamp examination and fluorescein angiography are required [3]. The only definite proof of ischemic RVO is the occurrence of neovascular complications, including vascular proliferation, vitreous hemorrhage, rubeosis iridis and secondary (neovascular) glaucoma ('100-day glaucoma'). Typically, venous filling is delayed (>20 s) by fluorescein angiography. Retinal neovascularization only occurs in the ischemic type of RVO in an estimated two thirds of cases. It has been shown to occur in 36% of eyes with a non-perfusion area larger than 5 optic disc diameters [1, 3].

Long-standing RVO are characterized by less or no residual intraretinal blood and resolution of cotton-wool spots. While there is less tortuositas of vessels in the affected segment, shunt vessels (collaterals) can frequently be seen. Macular edema can persist or may leave neurosensory atrophy with irregularities of the pigment epithelium after resorption.

Treatment of RVO

During the past decades, several treatment methods have been described for RVO. Most therapies focus on eliminating late complications and vision-disturbing effects of RVO. Overall, there is still only little evidence for the efficacy of specific treatment options due to lack of large randomized, prospective studies. In general, therapeutic strategies can be divided into acute interventions (within the first 3 months after RVO) and prophylactic measures aiming at reducing the risk of late complications. Besides, any underlying non-ocular disease should be diagnosed and treated, if possible. Because of the complex pathogenesis, treatment and prophylaxis of RVO is an interdisciplinary task and all patients with acute RVO should be referred to a specialist for internal medicine.

Acute Interventions
The aim of early therapeutic measures should be to improve the perfusion of the affected vessel and to reduce macular edema. Rheological therapy has long been considered to be the first-line treatment in acute RVO.

Rheological Therapy
Hemodilution can be performed as hyper- or isovolemic hemodilution. The latter can be controlled more easily and allows for significantly lower hematocrit values in the capillary bed. Isovolemic hemodilution is performed by simultaneous venesection and replacement of the lost volume by a plasma substitute, usually hydroxyethyl starch or dextran, leading to reduced blood viscosity and improving retinal blood flow [25]. Several authors described significantly better visual outcomes in treated patients [22–24]. However, these results have been discussed controversially because of the small study populations and because combined therapies were applied in some of the studies. Nevertheless, isovolemic hemodilution is accepted by several specialists as a first-line treatment within the first 8 weeks after BRVO, as it increases retinal perfusion and may prevent capillary closure and progressive retinal ischemia. The therapy is usually well tolerated; side effects include headache, dyspnea, deep vein thrombosis and hypotension [16]. Nevertheless, patients have to be carefully selected and should not have any severe cardiorespiratory or renal disease. Early treatment seems to be important in order to reduce the risk of subsequent ischemic complications. Late treatment does not seem to influence ischemia or prevent secondary glaucoma, therefore eyes showing established neovascularization will need additional laser coagulation [25].

Other rheologically active substances which have been tested for treatment of RVO include troxerutin and pentoxifylline. The first is thought to improve microcirculation in capillaries and venules by inhibiting erythrocyte and platelet aggregation improving erythrocyte deformability [26]. Pentoxifylline leads to vessel dilation and improves retinal flow [27]. Both substances have been used in the treatment of peripheral vein occlusions of the extremities. The efficacy of these drugs in patients with RVO has not sufficiently been proven in prospective studies yet.

Thrombolytic and Coagulation-Inhibiting Therapy

Currently there is only one randomized study comparing the effect of dalteparin and acetylsalicylate in patients with BRVO. No difference was found between the two anticoagulants. Apart from this study, no randomized clinical studies have been published concerning *systemic* treatment of BRVO with acetylsalicylate, heparin or intravasal thrombolysis with tissue plasminogen activator (rTPA). None of these treatments has been proven to be effective in the treatment of CRVO, and some of them have severe side effects when being used systemically [28]. One recently published study found a positive effect of systemic treatment of CRVO and BRVO with low-dose rTPA but no preventive effect concerning neovascularization [29]. Another case series found increased visual acuity after systemic treatment of RVOs with enoxaparin, a low-molecular-weight heparin [30].

Local thrombolysis with rTPA – either by intravitreal injection or, during vitreoretinal surgery, by direct injection into the occluded vessel – has been shown to be effective in patients with CRVO [31, 32]; currently there are no studies on its effectiveness in BRVO. However, treatment with rTPA has serious risks and was associated with complications, including vitreous hemorrhage and increase in macular edema [25, 28]. Its application is therefore very limited.

One study found a significant effect of the platelet aggregation inhibitor ticlopidine on visual acuity when administered within the first 3 weeks after vein occlusion and for a period of 6 months [33]. In general, anticoagulants should not be used without underlying coagulopathy and are contraindicated at the early stage because of the increased risk of subretinal bleedings.

Laser Treatment

Macular grid laser photocoagulation has been shown to be effective and is a commonly used method in patients with RVO. Many studies have been published, investigating different methods of laser coagulation, mainly macular grid-pattern laser for treatment of macular edema and peripheral scatter laser photocoagulation for prophylaxis and treatment of neovascularization. The clinical results vary largely between the different studies. The largest randomized, prospective trial (Branch Vein Occlusion Study Group) showed a positive effect of central grid laser on visual acuity in patients with BRVO [1]. However, other studies found no significant benefit for patients after central grid laser [34, 35]. In CRVO, grid laser photocoagulation was shown to decrease macular edema angiographically but not to improve visual acuity in patients with persistent macular edema [2]. It has therefore been largely abandoned for macular edema secondary to CRVO. However, grid laser treatment may be used in BRVO to treat a macular edema, which persists longer than 3–6 months or with serous retinal detachment [1, 36]. If fluorescein angiography shows macular non-perfusion, the effect of grid laser therapy is not guaranteed [1]. Grid laser treatment has been shown to be more effective in combination with intravitreal injections of TA in one study [56]. An argon laser was used by most authors. Grid laser treatment usually is not effective in RVO older than 1 year and in eyes with a VA of 20/200 or worse [37].

Peripheral scatter laser photocoagulation in ischemic (non-perfusion) areas significantly reduces the risk of retinal neovascularization and vitreous hemorrhage [2, 38]. The effectiveness of peripheral laser coagulation was demonstrated for eyes with non-perfusion areas, but also for eyes already showing neovascularization. However, the effect was greater when treatment was performed early, before neovascularization had developed. On the other hand, there are important side effects of scatter laser coagulation, primarily visual field defects. For that reason it has been proposed to wait with laser treatment until the first signs of neovascularization are clinically visible [38].

Another method, which has been suggested by several authors, is to create an anastomosis between a retinal vein and the choroid. This can be achieved by a neodymium yttrium-aluminum garnet (Nd:YAG) laser spot following intense argon laser treatment of a retinal vein segment [39]. Alternatively, it can be performed intraoperatively during vitrectomy, using an erbium:YAG laser [40]. Success rates of up to 54% have been reported, however a complication rate of 20% has also been described for laser-induced chorioretinal anastomosis.

Surgical Methods

The aim (and theoretical advantage) of surgical treatment of RVO is to remove the occlusion itself and to restore normal retinal blood flow. One method, which has been employed by several authors, is arteriovenous dissection (sheathotomy). Its purpose is to dissect the retinal artery from the adjacent vein in the area surrounding the vascular occlusion [41]. The procedure requires vitrectomy, followed by an incision of the adventitial sheath adjacent to the arteriovenous crossing and separation of the adhesions. Several studies have shown a positive effect of sheathotomy on visual acuity [41–49]. Different surgical techniques were used and surgery was combined with additional application of intravitreal triamcinolone, tissue plasminogen activator or other treatment methods in some of these (non-randomized) studies. Therefore, the effect of sheathotomy alone remains unclear. One study found no advantage of sheathotomy over treatment of BRVO with intravitreal TA [43].

The vitreous and the intact vitreoretinal surface are supposed to play a role in the development of neovascularization [25]. It has been postulated that vitrectomy alone with surgical detachment of the posterior hyaloid may be more relevant for the positive effect on visual acuity than arteriovenous dissection itself [45, 46, 50]. One study found no advantage of sheathotomy over sole vitrectomy [45]. Another study found no advantage of combined vitrectomy and intravitreal TA over vitrectomy alone [51].

An alternative surgical method which has been shown to improve visual acuity after RVO with persisting macular edema, is combined vitrectomy and peeling of the internal limiting membrane [52–54]. However, because of the lack of randomized prospective studies, the rationale why vitreoretinal surgery reduces the symptoms of BRVO remains unclear.

Corticosteroids

Corticosteroids lead to reduced permeability of the affected retinal vasculature and offer an anti-inflammatory and angiostatic effect, therefore reducing macular edema and the associated chronic damage to photoreceptors [55]. Several studies have shown a positive effect of intravitreal injections of triamcinolone acetonide (TA) [56–68]. In vitro, corticosteroids also inhibit VEGF expression and may thus prevent neovascularization and reduce the VEGF-mediated increase in retinal capillary permeability [25]. Unfortunately, most of the clinical studies were not randomized or did not distinguish between different types (ischemic/non-ischemic) of RVO. Some studies found a superior effect of combined intravitreal TA and macular grid laser photocoagulation therapy on visual acuity [56, 69, 70]. However, the positive anti-edematous effect of TA seems to be temporary, and several retreatments are usually necessary to avoid reoccurrence of macular edema and associated loss in visual acuity. The repetitive application in turn raises the risk for side effects of the treatment, mainly increased intraocular pressure, cataract progression and endophthalmitis [71–73]. Early treatment seems to be important, because chronic macular edema with persistence beyond 1 year often does not respond well to the treatment with intravitreal steroids or does not lead to an increase in visual acuity [25].

For a longer lasting therapeutic effect, the implantation of an intravitreous dexamethasone delivery system (Posurdex) has also been shown to be effective in the treatment of BRVO [74]. The side effects, mainly intraocular pressure rise, are similar to repeated intravitreal injections of TA. Another intraocular slow-release device is already approved in the USA and approval by the European authorities is pending.

Some effects on visual acuity have also been shown for retrobulbar injections of TA [67, 75–78], however these were less reliable than after intravitreal application of TA. Systemic application of steroids has also been reported to reduce macular edema and improve visual acuity, but should – because of the possible side effects – only be considered for younger patients with concurrent papillary edema or with an inflammatory component, especially in patients with systemic vasculitic disorder. However, currently there are only reports on the effectiveness of systemic steroid therapy in patients with CRVO [28], but no data regarding its potential usefulness in the treatment of BRVO.

Anti-VEGF Therapy

RVO leads to increased expression of VEGFs by retina and retinal pigment epithelium and an increased release into the vitreous, causing neovascularization, vascular hyperpermeability with subsequent breakdown of the blood retina barrier and thus macular edema. All three currently available VEGF inhibitors (ranibizumab, bevacizumab, pegaptanib) have been applied successfully in RVO. However, many prospective, randomized studies evaluating these agents against each other or a control group are still ongoing and the results have not been published yet. Therefore any use of anti-VEGF agents in this indication has to be considered as off-label. Most of the published studies used different doses (1.25–2.5 mg) of bevacizumab (Avastin®). In all of these series visual acuity increased and macular thickness was reduced for 3–9 weeks after the treatment [79]. However, most trials did not differentiate between different types of RVO. Recently, a number of studies focusing on the effect of bevacizumab on BRVO have been published, also demonstrating a significant increase in visual acuity and regression of the macular edema [80–90]. Encouraging results have also been published for anti-VEGF treatment of CRVO [79, 91–94]. It became obvious that not only central visual acuity, but also the overall retinal sensitivity improved significantly after anti-VEGF therapy [86]. One group demonstrated that patients who respond well to the initial injection of bevacizumab are most likely to achieve a long-term benefit from the treatment [85]. Two studies found a correlation between the intraocular VEGF concentrations and the severity of macular edema as well as a significant decrease of these factors in eyes treated with bevacizumab [95, 96]. Since central retinal thickness measurements correlated significantly with VEGF concentrations, optical coherence tomography (OCT) appears to offer an excellent biomarker for disease activity [95]. In many cases of recurrent macular edema after the first treatment, retreatment with bevacizumab again led to a reduction of the macular thickness. Altogether, there was a mean increase in visual acuity of more than three lines [16]. Similar results have been found for the treatment of BRVO with ranibizumab in the first published study [97]. In general, intravitreal treatment with VEGF inhibitors seems to have only a low risk of complications. The most common side effects include hyposphagma and conjunctival hyperemia. The disadvantage of anti-VEGF therapy is – similar to the treatment with corticosteroids – the short duration of the drug effect, usually requiring several retreatments to maintain the positive effects on macular edema and visual acuity. The effect of a single injection seems to last 6–8 weeks (fig. 1). Most authors used 2–3 injections over the first 5–6 months [80]. Also patients who do not respond well to laser therapy seem to benefit from intravitreal anti-VEGF therapy [80]. Two randomized, multicenter phase III studies of ranibizumab (Lucentis) (BRAVO study, CRUISE study) show early and sustained improvement in vision in patients with BTVO and CRVO [Retina Congress 2009; publication pending]. However, the condition of central macular edema does not necessarily reflect the overall ischemic situation of the entire retina and despite the absence of clinically significant macular edema, neovascularization of the disc may occur and lead to vitreous hemorrhage. These neovascular complications appear to be retarded under anti-VEGF therapy, but may still occur with a prolonged pathogenetic development.

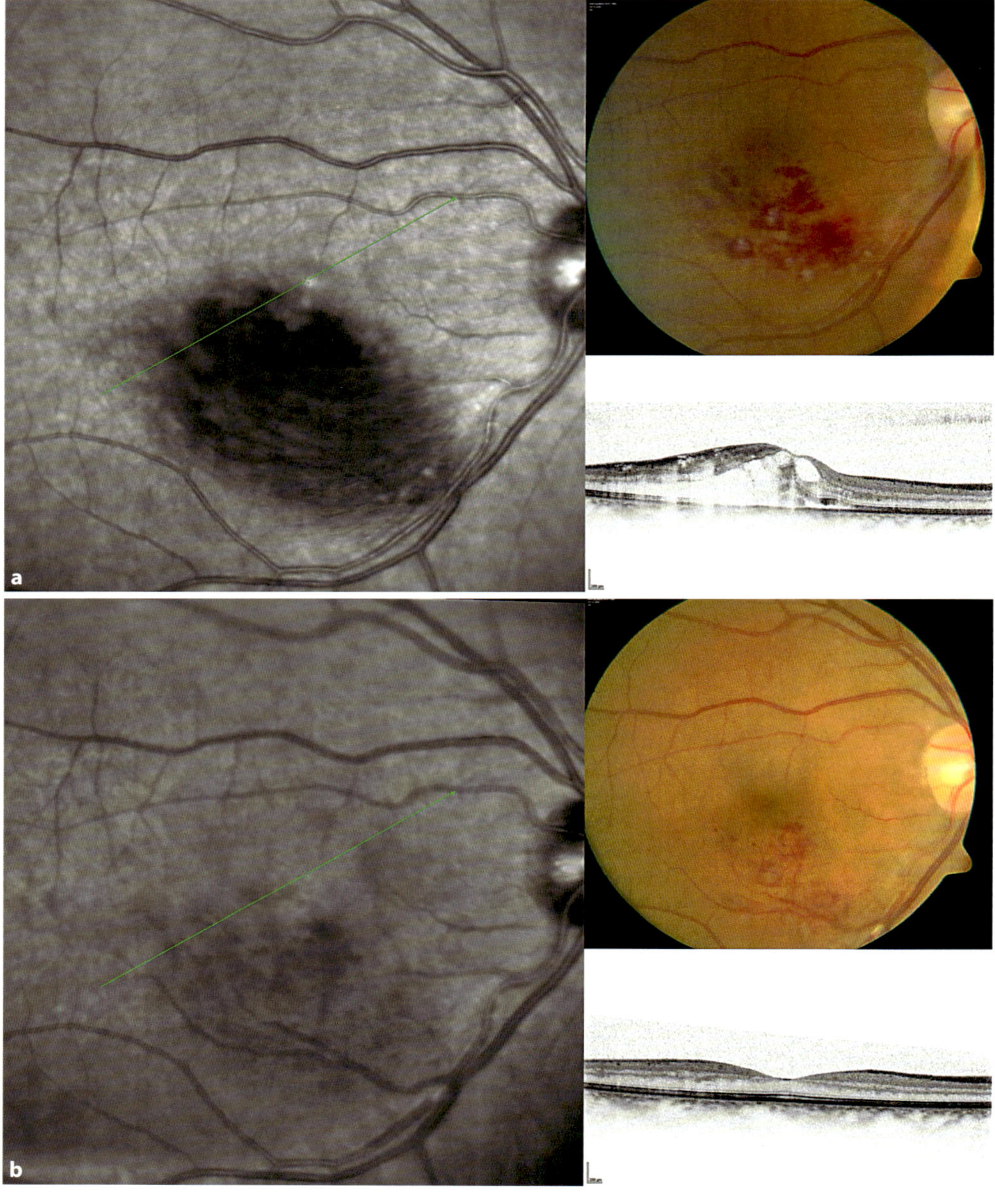

Fig. 1. Fundus and high-resolution OCT images of a patient with BRVO (**a**) before and (**b**) 2 months after treatment with ranibizumab (Lucentis®), showing resolution of bleedings and macular edema.

If given with appropriate timing, anti-VEGF treatment is also supposed to be effective in the treatment of the ischemic complications of RVO, reducing the risk of neovascularization and rubeosis iridis, and lowering intraocular pressure in neovascular glaucoma. This has already been shown in several publications on the effectiveness of anti-VEGF therapy in late complications of other retinal vascular diseases, mainly in diabetic retinopathy [98, 99]. Bevacizumab has also been applied intracamerally to successfully suppress neovascular glaucoma and rubeosis iridis [100].

Prophylactic Measures
In the late stadium of RVO the main focus should be directed to the prevention of secondary glaucoma. Ischemic areas larger than 5 optic disc diameters are associated with a distinctly increased risk of neovascular complications and should therefore be treated [1, 38]. Randomized studies have shown that peripheral scatter laser coagulation of non-perfusion areas can lead to a significant reduction of neovascular proliferations in those cases [38]. Consequently, follow-up examinations at short intervals are mandatory in all cases of RVO to detect non-perfusion areas in time. Future studies will have to show whether the use of anti-VEGF agents may perhaps replace the preventive effect of peripheral laser coagulation.

As mentioned before, prophylactic measures also include investigation and treatment of all associated risk factors, mainly arterial hypertension, diabetes mellitus, blood lipid and hematological disorders, in order to reduce the risk of a second event in the same or the contralateral eye.

Conclusion

Although several treatment methods for RVO have been shown to be effective, there is still a lack of large prospective, randomized studies for most therapies. The complex genesis of the disease with numerous risk factors and the variable progression, ranging from spontaneous recovery to exacerbation with severe ischemic complications, makes it difficult to find a common treatment scheme for BRVO. Laser coagulation is effective in the treatment of macular edema and neovascularization, but not in all cases, and it has significant functional side effects. Favorable results were also found for treatment with intravitreal triamcinolone; however, the effect is temporary and associated with severe ocular side effects. The approval of slow-release implants may improve the prospective of this strategy. The results for surgical treatment of RVO lack sufficient evidence, are largely variable and not appropriated per se to be applied in larger populations. The recently published data on intravitreal treatment with anti-VEGF substances is encouraging and gives hope for a further step ahead in the treatment of this frequent sight-threatening disease. Further studies will have to show whether the positive short-term effects of anti-VEGF therapy on macular edema and visual performance are only transient or may finally lead to a long-lasting stabilization and persistent improvement in visual acuity. The main problem is the short therapeutic effect of a single intravitreal injection. However, in contrast to other substances such as intravitreal TA, treatment with VEGF inhibitors has been shown to have remarkably few side effects even after many repeated injections. Perhaps combination of anti-VEGF therapy with other forms of treatment may reduce the number of required intravitreal injections. Prospective randomized trials evaluating different compounds and different regimen are ongoing. With respect to the multifactorial pathophysiology, including vascular and hematologic events as well as angiogenic and inflammatory stimuli, and the chronic nature of the disease, combined approaches may be required for an optimized management.

References

1 Branch Vein Occlusion Study Group: Argon laser photocoagulation for macular edema in branch vein occlusion. Am J Ophthalmol 1984;98:271–282.

2 Central Vein Occlusion Study Group: Natural history and clinical management of central retinal vein occlusion. Arch Ophthalmol 1997;115:486–491.

3 Parodi MB, Bandello F: Branch retinal vein occlusion: classification and treatment. Ophthalmologica 2009;223:298–305.

4 Klein R, Klein BE, Moss SE, Meuer SM: The epidemiology of retinal vein occlusion: the Beaver Dam Eye Study. Trans Am Ophthalmol Soc 2000;98:133–141.

5 Noma H, Funatsu H, Yamasaki M, et al: Pathogenesis of macular edema with branch retinal vein occlusion and intraocular levels of vascular endothelial growth factor and interleukin-6. Am J Ophthalmol 2005;140:256–261.

6 Kumar B, Yu DY, Morgan WH, Barry CJ, Constable IJ, McAllister IL: The distribution of angioarchitectural changes within the vicinity of the arteriovenous crossing in branch retinal vein occlusion. Ophthalmology 1998;105:424–427.

7 Mitchell P, Smith W, Chang A: Prevalence and associations of retinal vein occlusion in Australia. The Blue Mountains Eye Study. Arch Ophthalmol 1996; 114:1243–1247.

8 Cugati S, Wang JJ, Rochtchina E, Mitchell P: Ten-year incidence of retinal vein occlusion in an older population. The Blue Mountains Eye Study. Arch Ophthalmol 2006;124:726–732.

9 David R, Zangwill L, Badarna M, Yassur Y: Epidemiology of retinal vein occlusion and its association with glaucoma and increased intraocular pressure. Ophthalmologica 1998;197:69–74.

10 Bearelly S, Fekrat S: Controversy in the management of retinal venous occlusive disease. Int Ophthalmol Clin 2004;44:85–102.

11 Weinberg D, Dodwell DG, Fern SA: Anatomy of arteriovenous crossings in branch retinal vein occlusion. Am J Ophthalmol 1990;109:298–302.

12 Scott IU: Vitreoretinal surgery for complications of branch retinal vein occlusion. Curr Opin Ophthalmol 2002;13:161–166.

13 Feist RM, Ticho BH, Shapiro MJ, Farber M: Branch retinal vein occlusion and quadratic variation in arteriovenous crossings. Am J Ophthalmol 1992; 113:664–668.

14 Christoffersen NL, Larsen M: Pathophysiology and hemodynamics of branch retinal vein occlusion. Ophthalmology 1999;106:2054–2062.

15 Janssen MC, den Heijer M, Cruysberg JR, Wollersheim H, Bredie SJ: Retinal vein occlusion: a form of venous thrombosis or a complication of atherosclerosis? A meta-analysis of thrombophilic factors. Thromb Haemost 2005;93:1021–1026.

16 Rehak J, Rehak M: Branch retinal vein occlusion: pathogenesis, visual prognosis, and treatment modalities. Curr Eye Res 2008;33:111–131.

17 Ingerslev J: Thrombophilia: a feature of importance in retinal vein thrombosis? Acta Ophthalmol Scand 1999;77:619–621.

18 Tekeli O, Gürsel E, Buyurgan H: Protein C, protein S and antithrombin III deficiencies in retinal vein occlusion. Acta Ophthalmol Scand 1999;77:628–630.

19 Tost F: Venous branch occlusion due to APC resistance. Ophthalmologe 1999;96:777–780.

20 Hayreh SS: Prevalent misconceptions about acute retinal vascular occlusive disorders. Prog Retin Eye Res 2005;24:493–519.

21 Barbazetto IA, Schmidt-Erfurth UM: Evaluation of functional defects in branch retinal vein occlusion before and after laser treatment with scanning laser perimetry. Ophthalmology 2000;107:1089–1098.

22 Chen HC, Wiek J, Gupta A, et al: Effect of isovolaemic haemodilution on visual outcome in branch retinal vein occlusion. Br J Ophthalmol 1998;82:162–167.

23 Hansen LL, Wiek J, Arntz R: Randomized study of the effect of isovolemic hemodilution in retinal branch vein occlusion (in German). Fortschr Ophthalmol 1988;85:514–516.

24 Poupard P, Eledjam JJ, Dupeyron G, et al: Role of acute normovolemic hemodilution in treating retinal venous occlusions (in French). Ann Fr Anesth Reanim 1986;5:229–233.
25 Shahid H, Hossain P, Amoaku WM: The management of retinal vein occlusion: is interventional ophthalmology the way forward? Br J Ophthalmol 2006;90:627–639.
26 Glacet-Bernard A, Coscas G, Chabanel A, et al: A randomized, double-masked study on the treatment of retinal vein occlusion with troxerutin. Am J Ophthalmol 1994;118:421–429.
27 De Sanctis MT, Cesarone MR, Belcaro G, et al: Treatment of retinal vein thrombosis with pentoxifylline: a controlled, randomized trial. Angiology 2002;53(suppl 1):35–38.
28 Sharma A, D'Amico DJ: Medical and surgical management of central retinal vein occlusion. Int Ophthalmol Clin 2004;44:1–16.
29 Hattenbach LO, Friedrich Arndt C, Lerche R, et al: Retinal vein occlusion and low-dose fibrinolytic therapy: a prospective, randomized, controlled multicenter study of low-dose recombinant tissue plasminogen activator versus hemodilution in retinal vein occlusion. Retina 2009;29:932–940.
30 Steigerwalt RD Jr, Cesarone MR, Belcaro G, et al: Retinal and orbital venous occlusions treated with enoxaparin. J Ocul Pharmacol Ther 2008;24:421–426.
31 Lahey JM, Fong DS, Kearney J: Intravitreal tissue plasminogen activator for acute central retinal vein occlusion. Ophthalmic Surg Lasers 1999;30;427–434.
32 Weiss JN, Bynoe LA: Injection of tissue plasminogen activator into a branch retinal vein in eyes with central retinal vein occlusion. Ophthalmology 2001; 108:2249–2257.
33 Houtsmuller AJ, Vermeulen JA, Klompe M, et al: The influence of ticlopidine on the natural course of retinal vein occlusion. Agents Actions Suppl 1984; 15:219–229.
34 Parodi MB, Saviano S, Bergamini L, Ravalico G: Grid laser treatment of macular edema in macular branch retinal vein occlusion. Doc Ophthalmol 1999;97:427–431.
35 Parodi MB, Saviano S, Ravalico G: Grid laser treatment in macular branch retinal vein occlusion. Graefes Arch Clin Exp Ophthalmol 1999;237:1024–1027.
36 Parodi MB, DI Stefano G, Ravalico G: Grid laser treatment for exudative retinal detachment secondary to ischemic branch retinal vein occlusion. Retina 2008;28:97–102.
37 McIntosh RL, Mohamed Q, Saw SM, Wong TY: Interventions for branch retinal vein occlusion: an evidence-based systematic review. Ophthalmology 2007;114:835–846.
38 Branch Vein Occlusion Study Group: Argon laser scatter photocoagulation for prevention of neovascularization and hemorrhage in branch vein occlusion. Arch Ophthalmol 1986;104:34–41.
39 McAllister IL, Douglas JP, Constable IJ, et al: Laser-induced chorioretinal venous anastomosis for nonischemic central retinal vein occlusion: evaluation of the complications and their risk factors. Am J Ophthalmol 1998;126:219–229.
40 Quiroz-Mercado H, Sanchez-Buenfil E, Guerrero-Naranjo JL, et al: Successful erbium: YAG laser-induced chorioretinal venous anastomosis for the management of ischemic central retinal vein occlusion. A report of two cases. Graefes Arch Clin Exp Ophthalmol 2001;239:872–875.
41 Osterloh MD, Charles S: Surgical decompression of branch retinal vein occlusions. Arch Ophthalmol 1988,106:1469–1471.
42 Chung EJ, Freeman WR, Koh HJ: Visual acuity and multifocal electroretinographic changes after arteriovenous crossing sheathotomy for macular edema associated with branch retinal vein occlusion. Retina 2008,28:220–225.
43 Chung EJ, Lee H, Koh HJ: Arteriovenous crossing sheathotomy versus intravitreal triamcinolone acetonide injection for treatment of macular edema associated with branch retinal vein occlusion. Graefes Arch Clin Exp Ophthalmol 2008;246:967–974.
44 Garcia-Arumi J, Martinez-Castillo V, Boixadera A, Blasco H, Corcostegui B: Management of macular oedema in branch retinal vein occlusion with sheathotomy and recombinant tissue plasminogen activator. Retina 2004;24:530–540.
45 Yamamoto S, Saito W, Yagi F, Takeuchi S, Sato E, Mizunoya S: Vitrectomy with or without arteriovenous adventitial sheathotomy for macular edema associated with branch retinal vein occlusion. Am J Ophthalmol 2004;138:907–914.
46 Kumagai K, Furukawa M, Ogino N, Uemura A, Larson E: Long-term outcomes of vitrectomy with or without arteriovenous sheathotomy in branch retinal vein occlusion. Retina 2007;27:49–54.
47 Avci R, Inan U, Kaderli B: Evaluation of arteriovenous crossing sheathotomy for decompression of branch retinal vein occlusion. Eye 2008;22:120–127.
48 Horio N, Horiguchi M: Effect of arteriovenous sheathotomy on retinal blood flow and macular edema in patients with branch retinal vein occlusion. Am J Ophthalmol 2005;139:739–740.

49 Mason J, Feist R, White M Jr, Swanner J, McGwin G Jr, Emond T: Sheathotomy to decompress branch retinal vein occlusion: a matched control study. Ophthalmology 2004;111:540–545.
50 Han DP, Bennett SR, Williams DF, Dev S: Arteriovenous crossing dissection without separation of the retina vessels for treatment of branch retinal vein occlusion. Retina 2003;23:145–151.
51 Uemura A, Yamamoto S, Sato E, Sugawara T, Mitamura Y, Mizunoya S: Vitrectomy alone versus vitrectomy with simultaneous intravitreal injection of triamcinolone for macular edema associated with branch retinal vein occlusion. Ophthalmic Surg Lasers Imaging 2009;40:6–12.
52 Ma J, Yao K, Zhang Z, Tang X: 25-Gauge vitrectomy and triamcinolone acetonide-assisted internal limiting membrane peeling for chronic cystoid macular edema associated with branch retinal vein occlusion. Retina 2008;28:947–956.
53 Mandelcorn MS, Nrusimhadevara RK: Internal limiting membrane peeling for decompression of macular edema in retinal vein occlusion: a report of 14 cases. Retina 2004;24:348–355.
54 Mandelcorn MS, Mandelcorn E, Guan K, Adatia FA: Surgical macular decompression for macular edema in retinal vein occlusion. Can J Ophthalmol 2007;42:116–122.
55 McAllister IL, Vijayasekaran S, Chen SD, Yu DY: Effect of triamcinolone acetonide on vascular endothelial growth factor and occludin levels in branch retinal vein occlusion. Am J Ophthalmol 2009;147: 838–846.
56 SCORE Study Research Group: A randomized trial comparing the efficacy and safety of intravitreal triamcinolone with standard care to treat vision loss associated with macular edema secondary to branch retinal vein occlusion: The Standard Care vs. Corticosteroid for Retinal Vein Occlusion (SCORE) Study Report 6. Arch Ophthalmol 2009;127:1115–1128.
57 Avitabile T, Longo A, Reibaldi A: Intravitreal triamcinolone compared with macular laser grid photocoagulation for the treatment of cystoid macular edema. Am J Ophthalmol 2005;140:695–702.
58 Ozkiris A, Evereklioglu C, Erkilic K, Dogan H: Intravitreal triamcinolone acetonide for treatment of persistent macular edema in branch retinal vein occlusion. Eye 2007;20:13–17.
59 Jonas JB, Akkoyun I, Kamppeter B, Kreissig I, Degenring RF: Branch retinal vein occlusion treated by intravitreal triamcinolone acetonide. Eye 2005; 19:65–71.
60 Cekic O, Chang S, Tseng JJ, et al: Intravitreal triamcinolone injection for treatment of macular edema secondary to branch retinal vein occlusion. Retina 2005;25:851–855.
61 Lee H, Shah GK: Intravitreal triamcinolone as primary treatment of cystoid macular edema secondary to branch retinal vein occlusion. Retina 2005; 25:551–555.
62 Yepremyan M, Wertz FD, Tivnan T, Eversman L, Marx JL: Early treatment of cystoid macular edema secondary to branch retinal vein occlusion with intravitreal triamcinolone acetonide. Ophthalmic Surg Lasers Imaging 2005;36:30–36.
63 Chen SD, Sundaram V, Lochhead J, Patel CK: Intravitreal triamcinolone for the treatment of ischemic macular edema associated with branch retinal vein occlusion. Am J Ophthalmol 2006;141:876–883.
64 Karacorlu M, Ozdemir H, Karacorlu SA: Resolution of serous macular detachment after intravitreal triamcinolone acetonide treatment of patients with branch retinal vein occlusion. Retina 2005;25:856–860.
65 Roth DB, Cukras C, Radhakrishnan R, et al: Intravitreal triamcinolone acetonide injections in the treatment of retinal vein occlusions. Ophthalmic Surg Lasers Imaging 2008;39:446–454.
66 Cakir M, Dogan M, Bayraktar Z, et al: Efficacy of intravitreal triamcinolone for the treatment of macular edema secondary to branch retinal vein occlusion in eyes with or without grid laser photocoagulation. Retina 2008;28:465–472.
67 Patel PJ, Zaheer I, Karia N: Intravitreal triamcinolone acetonide for macular oedema owing to retinal vein occlusion. Eye 2008;22:60–64.
68 Ozdek S, Deren YT, Gurelik G, Hasanreisoglu B: Posterior subtenon triamcinolone, intravitreal triamcinolone and grid laser photocoagulation for the treatment of macular edema in branch retinal vein occlusion. Ophthalmic Res 2008;40:26–31.
69 Riese J, Loukopoulos V, Meier C, Timmermann M, Gerding H: Combined intravitreal triamcinolone injection and laser photocoagulation in eyes with persistent macular edema after branch retinal vein occlusion. Graefes Arch Clin Exp Ophthalmol 2008; 246:1671–1676.
70 Parodi MB, Iacono P, Ravalico G: Intravitreal triamcinolone acetonide combined with subthreshold grid laser treatment for macular oedema in branch retinal vein occlusion: a pilot study. Br J Ophthalmol 2008;92:1046–1050.
71 Jonas JB, Degenring RF, Kreissig I, Akkoyun I, Kamppeter BA: Intraocular pressure elevation after intravitreal triamcinolone acetonide injection. Ophthalmology 2005;112:593–598.
72 Jonas JB, Degenring RF, Kreissig I, Akkoyun I: Safety of intravitreal high-dose reinjections of triamcinolone acetonide. Am J Ophthalmol 2004;138: 1054–1055.

73 Scott IU, Flynn HW Jr: Reducing the risk of endophthalmitis following intravitreal injections. Retina 2007;27:10–12.

74 Kuppermann BD, Blumenkranz MS, Haller JA, et al: Dexamethasone DDS Phase II Study Group: Randomized controlled study of an intravitreous dexamethasone drug delivery system in patients with persistent macular edema. Arch Ophthalmol 2007; 125:309–317.

75 Kawaji T, Takano A, Inomata Y, et al: Trans-Tenon's retrobulbar triamcinolone acetonide injection for macular oedema related to branch retinal vein occlusion. Br J Ophthalmol 2008;92:81–83.

76 Kawaji T, Hirata A, Awai N, et al: Trans-Tenon retrobulbar triamcinolone injection for macular edema associated with branch retinal vein occlusion remaining after vitrectomy. Am J Ophthalmol 2005; 140:540–542.

77 Hayashi K, Hayashi H: Intravitreal versus retrobulbar injections of triamcinolone for macular edema associated with branch retinal vein occlusion. Am J Ophthalmol 2005;139:972–982.

78 Wakabayashi T, Okada AA, Morimura Y, et al: Trans-Tenon retrobulbar triamcinolone infusion for chronic macular edema in central and branch retinal vein occlusion. Retina 2004;24:964–967.

79 Prager F, Michels S, Kriechbaum K, et al: Intravitreal bevacizumab (Avastin) for macular oedema secondary to retinal vein occlusion: 12-month results of a prospective clinical trial. Br J Ophthalmol 2009; 93:452–456.

80 Badalà F: The treatment of branch retinal vein occlusion with bevacizumab. Curr Opin Ophthalmol 2008;19:234–238.

81 Gregori NZ, Rattan GH, Rosenfeld PJ, et al: Safety and efficacy of intravitreal bevacizumab (Avastin) for the management of branch and hemiretinal vein occlusion. Retina 2009;29:913–925.

82 Ahmadi AA, Chuo JY, Banashkevich A, Ma PE, Maberley DA: The effects of intravitreal bevacizumab on patients with macular edema secondary to branch retinal vein occlusion. Can J Ophthalmol 2009;44:154–159.

83 Jaissle GB, Leitritz M, Gelisken F, Ziemssen F, Bartz-Schmidt KU, Szurman P: One-year results after intravitreal bevacizumab therapy for macular edema secondary to branch retinal vein occlusion. Graefes Arch Clin Exp Ophthalmol 2009;247:27–33.

84 Abegg M, Tappeiner C, Wolf-Schnurrbusch U, Barthelmes D, Wolf S, Fleischhauer J: Treatment of branch retinal vein occlusion induced macular edema with bevacizumab. BMC Ophthalmol 2008; 29:8–18.

85 Chung EJ, Hong YT, Lee SC, Kwon OW, Koh HJ: Prognostic factors for visual outcome after intravitreal bevacizumab for macular edema due to branch retinal vein occlusion. Graefes Arch Clin Exp Ophthalmol 2008;246:1241–1247.

86 Kriechbaum K, Michels S, Prager F, et al: Intravitreal Avastin for macular oedema secondary to retinal vein occlusion: a prospective study. Br J Ophthalmol 2008;92:518–522.

87 Kreutzer TC, Alge CS, Wolf AH, et al: Intravitreal bevacizumab for the treatment of macular oedema secondary to branch retinal vein occlusion. Br J Ophthalmol 2008;92:351–355.

88 Wu L, Arevalo JF, Roca JA, et al: Pan-American Collaborative Retina Study Group (PACORES): Comparison of two doses of intravitreal bevacizumab (Avastin) for treatment of macular edema secondary to branch retinal vein occlusion: results from the Pan-American Collaborative Retina Study Group at 6 months of follow-up. Retina 2008;28:212–219.

89 Rabena MD, Pieramici DJ, Castellarin AA, Nasir MA, Avery RL: Intravitreal bevacizumab (Avastin) in the treatment of macular edema secondary to branch retinal vein occlusion. Retina 2007;27:419–425.

90 Spandau U, Wickenhauser A, Rensch F, Jonas J: Intravitreal bevacizumab for branch retinal vein occlusion. Acta Ophthalmol Scand 2007;85:118–119.

91 Stahl A, Struebin I, Hansen LL, Agostini HT, Feltgen N: Bevacizumab in central retinal vein occlusion: a retrospective analysis after 2 years of treatment. Eur J Ophthalmol 2010;20:180–185.

92 Guthoff R, Meigen T, Hennemann K, Schrader W: Comparison of bevacizumab and triamcinolone for treatment of macular edema secondary to central retinal vein occlusion – a matched-pairs analysis. Ophthalmologica 2010;224:126–132.

93 Gregori NZ, Gaitan J, Rosenfeld PJ, Puliafito CA, Feuer W, Flynn HW Jr, Berrocal AM, Al-Attar L, Dubovy S, Smiddy WE, Schwartz SG, Lee WH, Murray TG: Long-term safety and efficacy of intravitreal bevacizumab (Avastin) for the management of central retinal vein occlusion. Retina 2008;28: 1325–1337.

94 Wu WC, Cheng KC, Wu HJ: Intravitreal triamcinolone acetonide vs. bevacizumab for treatment of macular oedema due to central retinal vein occlusion. Eye 2009;23:2215–2222.

95 Funk M, Kriechbaum K, Prager F, et al: Intraocular concentrations of growth factors and cytokines in retinal vein occlusion and the effect of therapy with bevacizumab. Invest Ophthalmol Vis Sci 2009;50: 1025–1032.

96 Park SP, Ahn JK: Changes of aqueous vascular endothelial growth factor and pigment epithelium-derived factor following intravitreal bevacizumab for macular oedema secondary to branch retinal vein occlusion. Clin Exp Ophthalmol 2009;37:490–495.
97 Campochiaro PA, Hafiz G, Shah SM, et al: Ranibizumab for macular edema due to retinal vein occlusions: implication of VEGF as a critical stimulator. Mol Ther 2008;16:791–799.
98 Iliev ME, Domig D, Wolf-Schnurrbursch U, Wolf S, Sarra GM: Intravitreal bevacizumab (Avastin) in the treatment of neovascular glaucoma. Am J Ophthalmol 2006;142:1054–1056.
99 Yazdani S, Hendi K, Pakravan M: Intravitreal bevacizumab (Avastin) injection for neovascular glaucoma. J Glaucoma 2007;16:437–439.
100 Grisanti S, Biester S, Peters S, Tatar O, Ziemssen F, Bartz-Schmidt KU: Tübingen Bevacizumab Study Group: Intracameral bevacizumab for iris rubeosis. Am J Ophthalmol 2006;142:158–160.

Prof. Ursula Schmidt-Erfurth
Department of Ophthalmology and Optometry
Medical University Vienna
Waehringer Guertel 18-20, AT–1090 Vienna (Austria)
E-Mail ursula.schmidt-erfurth@meduniwien.ac.at

Bandello F, Battaglia Parodi M (eds): Anti-VEGF.
Dev Ophthalmol. Basel, Karger, 2010, vol 46, pp 73–83

Antivascular Endothelial Growth Factor for Choroidal Neovascularization in Pathologic Myopia

Maurizio Battaglia Parodi[a] · Pierluigi Iacono[b] · Francesco Bandello[a]

[a]Department of Ophthalmology, University Vita-Salute, Scientific Institute San Raffaele, Milan, and [b]Fondazione G.B. Bietti per l'Oftalmologia, Istituto di Ricovero e Cura a Carattere Scientifico, Rome, Italy

Abstract

Choroidal neovascularization (CNV) is the most common vision-threatening macular complication in pathologic myopia (PM) being detectable in 4–11% of the affected eyes. Treatment of PM-related CNV is still controversial. Intravitreal injections of antivascular endothelial growth factor molecules are able to inhibit the vascular endothelial growth factor isoforms and have shown promise in the treatment of myopic CNV. The present review describes the beneficial effects of this approach both for subfoveal and juxtafoveal CNV. However, considering the lack of randomized clinical trials and the relatively short follow-up in most of the studies, a multicentric clinical trial should be necessary to validate the positive results in the long term.

Pathologic myopia (PM) represents one of the major causes of legal blindness in many developed countries [1], presenting a prevalence of about 2% in the general population [2]. PM is defined as an eye having a minimum refractive error of –6 dpt, an axial length >26 mm, associated with degenerative changes of the retina, choroid and sclera at the posterior segment [3]. Common findings are posterior staphyloma, chorioretinal atrophy, and lacquer cracks in the Bruch's membrane [4]. Choroidal neovascularization (CNV) is the most common vision-threatening macular complication in PM [5], being detectable in 4–11% of the eyes affected by PM [2, 4, 5].

Myopic CNV has typical characteristics, such as small dimensions (usually less than 1 disc diameter), more often subfoveal or juxtafoveal location, complete absence or limited presence of subretinal fluid, hemorrhage, or hard exudates [4]. Moreover, myopic CNV has specific histopathological features being a type 2 CNV, which is situated between the sensory retina and retinal pigment epithelium (RPE), and is entirely coated by RPE. More specifically, PM-related CNV is characterized by a RPE layer on its inner surface and a RPE inverted layer on its outer surface, creating a twofold RPE layer [6].

Natural History

The long-term visual prognosis of subfoveal myopic CNV without treatment is poor, with a visual acuity of 20/200 or less after 5–10 years of follow-up [7]. In particular, the CNV tends to a progressive enlargement with fibrotic evolution, whereas chorioretinal atrophic changes develop around the myopic CNV especially in older patients [8–10]. It is noteworthy that patients under the age of 40 have significantly better visual outcome than patients over the age of 40 [9].

Less data are available regarding the natural history of juxtafoveal myopic CNV. A retrospective, observational study on 9 patients affected by juxtafoveal myopic CNV with a mean follow-up of 5.8 years has revealed that final visual acuity was 20/40 in 77% of the cases, but unfortunately the authors do not report the baseline VA values, making the interpretation of these data difficult [11]. The results have been confirmed by another investigation involving 11 eyes with juxtafoveal myopic CNV, which, after a follow-up of 5 years, showed a final VA <5/10 in 45% of the examined cases [12–15].

Treatment Options

Treatment of PM-related CNV is still controversial. During the past decades, laser photocoagulation has been the only effective means of treating non-subfoveal CNV associated with PM, but the functional outcome has turned out to be unsatisfactory in the long term. In the largest published study, the comparison of laser photocoagulation with the natural history showed laser-treated eyes to have a statistically better visual acuity at 2 years, but this difference was not statistically significant after 5 years of follow-up [16]. Such late failure is generally due to the typical expansion of the laser scar, which is seen in 90–100% of the treated eyes [16]. Two limited case series have reported positive results about photodynamic therapy (PDT) for juxtafoveal myopic CNV [17, 18].

Despite the relative positive effects of PDT in subfoveal myopic CNV demonstrated at 12 months by the VIP (Verteporfin in Photodynamic Therapy) study [19], the 2-year outcomes failed to reveal a statistically significant treatment benefit [20]. Alternative therapies like radiotherapy [21], surgical removal of the CNV [22] and macular translocation [23] have not been shown to be worth the collateral damage incurred by them.

In PM, mechanical tissue strain caused by axial length elongation may lead to the development of choroidal ischemia followed by atrophy of the RPE and overlying retina and subsequent vascular endothelial growth factor (VEGF) release [4]. The risk of developing CNV was, thus, found to be greatest in eyes with patchy atrophy or lacquer cracks [4]. Intravitreal injections of anti-VEGF molecules, such as bevacizumab and ranibizumab, are able to inhibit all the VEGF isoforms [24] and have shown promise in the treatment of myopic CNV.

Anti-VEGF for Myopic CNV

Several investigators have tried to assess the effects of intravitreal anti-VEGF administration for the treatment of myopic CNV reporting positive results [25–37]. Both naive CNV [25–30] and PDT-treated CNV [29–32] have been taken into consideration by a number of surveys. Subfoveal CNV has been analyzed by most of the studies, but some case series examined also cases presenting juxtafoveal CNV [25, 28, 32]. Intravitreal bevacizumab has been employed by the majority of the investigations [25–34], whereas only a few studies have made use of ranibizumab [35, 36].

Dosages used varied from 1 to 2.5 mg, and in general the protocol required a monthly injection for the first 3 months, followed by an as per needed injection for the subsequent period [25–36]. Overall, the anti-VEGF approach for PM-related CNV has been demonstrated to offer improved functional and anatomic advantages with respect to the previous treatment options, but all the studies available in the current literature are burdened by several limitations, including a limited number of patients, a short follow-up (3–12 months), the lack of a control group, the variability in the treatment protocol, and often the retrospective design of the analysis.

Subfoveal Myopic CNV

The results of VIP studies indicated that PDT-treated eyes were more likely to lose fewer than 8 letters (72%) than placebo-treated eyes (44%) after 1 year, 32% of treated eyes gaining at least 5 letters with respect to 15% of the placebo-treated eyes [19]. Unfortunately, the results were no longer statistically significant at the second year of follow-up [20]. Starting from these unsatisfactory results, several authors have reported interesting data about the use of anti-VEGF drugs in the treatment of PM-related subfoveal CNV.

All the studies have shown a visual acuity improvement over their follow-ups [25–37]. Nevertheless, a significant reduction of mean central macular thickness (CMT) was registered only by a few analyses [29, 30, 32, 37]. This optical coherence tomographic (OCT) feature seems to be a characteristic finding of myopic CNV, which generally show a mild degree of exudation [4]. All the studies have described reduction or stoppage of dye leakage on fluorescein angiography (FA) or CNV size reduction as an indication of response to therapy [25–37].

Interestingly, a single study has found that patients aged less and greater than 50 achieved a similar visual acuity improvement of about 8 letters [37], showing that intravitreal bevacizumab is effective also in older patients on the contrary to PDT, where 50% of older patients compared to 20% of younger patients lose at least 15 letters [38].

Our experience is related to a prospective, single-center, interventional case series with a planned follow-up of 2 years. 30 eyes of 30 patients were enrolled in the study.

Table 1. Inclusion and exclusion criteria for intravitreal bevacizumab in subfoveal myopic CNV

Inclusion criteria	Exclusion criteria
Subfoveal myopic CNV as delineated by FA	Intraocular surgery of any kind within 6 months of the day of injection
BCVA ≥20/400 and ≤20/32 on ETDRS chart	Significant media opacity likely to interfere with the measurement of BCVA
Previous PDT was allowed if performed at least 3 months prior to the day of injection	Prior history of ischemic heart disease or cerebral stroke
Females at least 12 months post-menopause or using standardized contraception if they are in the fertile age	Uncontrolled hypertension
Patients willing to sign a written, informed consent approved by the local IRB, and capable of adhering to the follow-up schedule	Pregnant and lactating women or women using non- standardized methods of contraception

Inclusion and exclusion criteria have been listed in table 1. 24 (80%) of the patients had received previous therapy with PDT (mean number of PDT sessions: 1.77). The injection procedure was performed in the operating room by an experienced retinologist under sterile precautions. Bevacizumab (1 mg/0.04 ml) was injected at the pars plana 3.5–4 mm from the surgical limbus in the inferotemporal quadrant using a 30-gauge needle and 1-ml syringe. The primary outcome measure was changed in mean best corrected visual acuity (BCVA) and proportion of eyes improving in BCVA by ≥3 lines. The secondary outcome measures included change in mean CMT, change in area of CNV, and proportion of eyes resolving in subretinal fluid/intraretinal fluid (SRF/IRF). Bevacizumab injections were given only on an as per needed basis as decided by CNV activity on FA and OCT. The follow-up visits were carried out on a monthly basis and included measurement of BCVA, OCT and FA.

Mean BCVA was 0.6 ± 0.3 at baseline, 0.54 ± 0.4 at the 12-month examination, and 0.50 ± 0.4 at the end of the follow-up, with no statistically significant difference (table 2). At the end of the follow-up, 11 eyes (36.6%) showed a BCVA improvement of 3 lines or greater. 13 eyes (43.3%) gained at least 1 line, while 11 (36.6%) showed a BCVA stabilization. On the other hand, 6 eyes (20%) lost at least 1 line of BCVA (table 3). Overall, mean CMT showed no statistically significant reduction from the baseline value (216.8 ± 86.7 μm) up to the end of 24 months (205 ± 77.8 μm) (table 2).

Even in the 11 out of 30 cases that showed visual improvement by 3 lines or greater, mean CMT showed no significant reduction ($p > 0.05$) at 24 months (188.4 ± 99.8 μm) from the baseline (179.7 ± 57.7 μm) or at any point in between. The only significant difference in CMT noted was between the baseline CMT in the group (179.7 ±

Table 2. Comparison of BCVA and CMT over the course of follow-up (mo = months)

Characteristic	Baseline	1 mo	3 mo	6 mo	12 mo	18 mo	24 mo
BCVA, logMAR (mean ± SD)	0.6 ±0.3	0.55 ±0.3	0.54 ±0.4	0.56 ±0.3	0.54 ±0.4	0.55 ±0.4	0.5 ±0.4
p value		0.003	0.91	0.78	0.47	0.67	1
CMT, μm (mean ± SD)	216.8 ±86.7	214.5 ±83.4	197 ±89.9	190 ±75.8	209 ±78.7	204 ±80.3	205 ±77.8
p value		0.8	0.48	0.53	0.18	0.32	0.82

Table 3. Comparison of baseline characteristics

Baseline characteristic	BCVA improvement by 3 lines or greater (n = 11)	BCVA stabilization or worsening by 3 lines or greater (n = 19)	p value
BCVA, logMAR (mean ± SD)	0.69±0.24	0.60±0.33	0.38
CMT, μm (mean ±SD)	179.7±57.7	276.3±94.5	0.044
Area of CNV, mm³ (mean ± SD)	1,370.4±1,223.3	3,743.5±3,659.5	0.016
Number of previous treatments (mean ± SD)	1.6 ±1.5	2.1±1.7	0.44
Presence of subretinal/ intraretinal fluid	4/11	10/19	0.46
Presence of subfoveal hemorrhage or scar	3/11	13/19	0.056
Age, years (mean ± SD)	57.9±11.6	62.1±12.5	0.37
Refractive error (mean ± SD)	−10.8±5.3	−9.9±5.1	0.64

57.7 μm) that improved in vision by at least 3 lines and the group (276.3 ± 94.5 μm) that remained stable in vision or worsened by at least 3 lines ($p = 0.044$) (table 3).

At baseline, 14 eyes (46.7%) presented with SRF/IRF. At 12 months, the cases with SRF/IRF decreased to 7 (23.3%), a non-significant ($p = 0.11$) difference compared to the baseline. However, at 24 months, the cases with SRF/IRF decreased to a mere 4 (13.3%), a significant ($p = 0.01$) difference compared to the baseline. In the 4 eyes with persistent SRF/IRF, fluid levels remained constant over at least the last 6 months of follow-up.

The area of CNV measured underwent a statistically significant reduction from baseline (2,873.4 ± 3,190.8 mm^3) to the 12-month examination (1,853.2 ± 2,174.6 mm^3), up

Table 4. Comparison of area of CNV over the course of follow-up

Characteristic	Baseline	3 months	12 months	18 months	24 months
Area of CNV, mm^3 (mean ± SD)	2,873.4 ±3,190.8	2,178.2 ±2,489.3	1,853.2 ±2,174.6	1,576.8 ±1,549.6	1,481.6 ±1,453
p value		0.08	0.001	0.16	0.12

to the 24-month examination (1,481.6 ± 1,453) (table 4). There was also a significant difference (p = 0.016) in baseline area of CNV noted between the group that improved in vision by 3 lines or greater (1,370 ± 1,223 mm^3) and the group that remained stable in vision or worsened by 3 lines or greater (3,743.5 ± 3,659.5 mm^3) (table 4). The mean number of IVB injections received was 4.13 over 24 months. No significant ocular or systemic adverse effects were registered over the course of the follow-up.

The present study demonstrates good functional results of intravitreal bevacizumab therapy for subfoveal myopic CNV in the long term. Our data compare favorably with respect to those of the VIP study. In particular, a BCVA improvement of 3 lines was registered in 36.6% of eyes in comparison with the 12% of VIP study. An intravitreal bevacizumab administration on as per needed basis can also remarkably reduce the number of injections, allowing a BCVA stabilization and a size reduction over a 2-year follow-up. The positive clinical outcomes need to be confirmed by means of a randomized clinical trial.

Juxtafoveal Myopic CNV

Limited data are available regarding the effects of anti-VEGF therapy for juxtafoveal myopic CNV. Sakaguchi et al. [25] reported on 2 eyes affected by juxtafoveal myopic CNV which achieved a functional and angiographic improvement after a single bevacizumab injection at the 4-month examination. Chan et al. [32] described 2 eyes with juxtafoveal CNV secondary to PM who underwent 3 monthly injections, reporting a visual acuity improvement with fibrotic evolution of the lesion at the 6-month examination. The study by Gharbiya et al. [28] included also subfoveal and juxtafoveal CNV, unfortunately not providing separate results for each subtype of CNV.

We designed a prospective randomized clinical trial to compare the effects of laser treatment (LT), PDT and intravitreal bevacizumab treatment in patients affected by juxtafoveal myopic CNV over a 24-month follow-up period. Inclusion and exclusion criteria are listed in table 5.

The recruited patients were divided into three subgroups: (1) *PDT group*, with subjects who underwent PDT with verteporfin; (2) *LT group*, including patients who

Table 5. Inclusion and exclusion criteria for the treatment of juxtafoveal myopic CNV

Inclusion criteria	Exclusion criteria
Classic, well-defined juxtafoveal myopic CNV (1–199 μm from the foveal center) evidenced on FA	Evidence of any condition other than myopia associated with CNV
Greatest linear dimension not more than 5,400 μm	Any significant ocular disease that had compromised or could compromise vision in the study eye
BCVA from 20/200 to 20/40 on ETDRS charts	Active hepatitis or clinically significant liver disease, porphyria or other porphyrin sensitivity, pregnancy, peripheral vascular disease, thromboembolism or stroke
Duration of symptoms inferior to 1 month	Intraocular surgery within the last 2 months or capsulotomy in the study eye within the last month
Documented visual acuity deterioration within the last month	Previous laser photocoagulation

underwent krypton laser photocoagulation of the JCNV, and (3) *Bevacizumab group*, including patients who underwent intravitreal bevacizumab injection (IVBI). Each patient was randomly allocated to one of the three treatment groups according to a computer-generated code number. Eyes in the LT group who developed recurrent CNV with subfoveal location over the follow-up period could be retreated using PDT.

The patients of the Bevacizumab group received intravitreal injections in the operating theater under sterile conditions. In particular, IVBI was performed 3.5–4.0 mm posterior to the corneal limbus using a 30-gauge needle after topical anesthesia. Additional IVBI were administered when the OCT examination revealed persistent or recurrent SR/IRF or when the FA examination revealed CNV activity or progression. The main outcome measure was the postoperative change in visual acuity compared with the baseline examination in all subgroups. 54 patients affected by JCNV in PM were recruited. 38 patients were females and 17 were males. 18 patients were randomized to PDT, 17 to LT, and 19 to IVBI. The demographic characteristics of the patients are outlined in table 6.

Table 7 shows mean BCVA in the three treatment arms during follow-up. At the baseline no statistically significant difference was registered among the three groups. At the 3- and 6-month follow-up, a substantial stabilization of the BCVA was observed in the LT and PDT group, whereas a statistically significant improvement was recorded in the IVBI group. At the 9-month follow-up, mean BCVA significantly

Table 6. Demographic characteristics of the patients randomized to LT, PDT and IVBI groups

	LT (17 eyes)	PDT (18 eyes)	IVBI (19 eyes)
Females	14 (82%)	13 (72%)	11 (57%)
Age	44.5	48.1	50.8
Diopters (SE)	−10.2	−9.2	−9.6
Hypertension	2 (11%)	2 (11%)	1 (5%)

Table 7. BCVA changes (logMAR) over the 24-month (mo) follow-up

	Baseline	3 mo	6 mo	9 mo	12 mo		18 mo	24 mo	
PDT group	0.52	0.51	0.49	0.67	0.67	$p < 0.05$ ↓	0.68	0.72	$p < 0.05$ ↓
LT group	0.45	0.46	0.41	0.39	0.47	NS vs. baseline	0.49	0.56	NS vs. baseline
				$p < 0.05$ vs. PDT	$p < 0.05$ vs. PDT		NS vs. PDT	NS vs. PDT	
IVBI	0.6	0.4	0.4	0.4	0.4	$p < 0.05$ ↑	0.42	0.42	$p < 0.05$ ↑
				$p < 0.05$ vs. PDT	$p < 0.05$ vs. PDT		$p < 0.05$ vs. PDT	$p < 0.05$ vs. PDT	

worsened to 0.67 in the PDT group ($p < 0.05$). At the same time, the LT group preserved initial visual acuity, and the IVBI group maintained the initial gain. At the 1-year follow-up, the PDT group showed a worsening of the mean BCVA with respect to the baseline. The LT group maintained the baseline mean BCVA, whereas only the IVBI group showed a statistically significant BCVA improvement. Moreover, a statistically significant difference favoring LT and IVBI versus PDT treatment was found at 9 and 12 months. At the 18- and 24-month follow-up visit, the IVBI group maintained the initial improvement in BCVA with a final gain of 1.8 lines from the baseline value to the 24-month examination value. The LT group showed a stabilization with respect to baseline with a visual loss not statistically significant of 1.1 lines, whereas the BCVA decreased in the PDT group from 0.52 at baseline to 0.72 at the end of the study with a statistically significant worsening of 2 lines. At the 24-month examination visit, only the Bevacizumab group had a statistically significant difference in comparison to the PDT group, with a mean difference of 3 lines. Table 8 summarizes the BCVA changes after the treatment in each subgroup. At the final

Table 8. Frequency distribution of changes in BCVA from baseline during the follow-up

	Lines gain/loss				
	≤3	≤1	0	>1	>3
PDT group	8 (44%)	13 (72%)	1 (5.5%)	4 (22%)	1(5.5%)
LT group	7 (41%)	10 (59%)	1 (6%)	6 (35%)	2 (12%)
Anti-VEGF group	1 (5%)	4 (21%)	2 (11%)	13 (68%)	7 (36%)

Table 9. PDT sessions and foveal extension of the juxtafoveal CNV registered in LT and PDT groups

		LT	PDT	Anti-VEGF
12 months	PDT sessions	0.6	2.3	excluded
	Foveal extension	9 (53%)	13 (72%)	4 (21%)
24 months	PDT sessions	0.5	1.2	excluded
	Foveal extension	0	0	0

visit, 5, 30 and 58% of PDT, LT, and IVBI groups, respectively, showed a BCVA better than 20/40.

The IVBI group showed the greater chance to preserve the initial BCVA or gain ETDRS lines (χ^2 test: $p < 0.005$). During the first year of follow-up, CNV recurrence with subfoveal extension was registered in 9 eyes (53%) in the LT group, which were retreated using PDT in accordance with the study protocol; a foveal extension developed in 13 eyes (72%) of the PDT group, whereas 4 eyes showed a CNV foveal extension in the IVBI group (table 9). Overall, 80% of subfoveal CNV recurrences occurred during the first 6 months of follow-up. No subfoveal CNV recurrence was detected in the second year.

The mean number of PDT sessions was 2.3 and 0.6 in the PDT and LT groups, respectively, during the first year of follow-up. The mean number of PDT treatments within the following 12 months of follow-up were 1.2 in the PDT group and 0.5 in the LT group. During the 24 months of follow-up, the mean number of IVBI was 3.8 ± 2.5, ranging between 1 and 11; only 4 patients required additional IVBI during the second year. Average mean CFT measured by OCT improved from 234 μm at baseline to 201 μm at the 1-month examination; this reduction was preserved up till 6 months and following a slight increase to 226 μm was recorded at the 12-month visit. In the second year, the assessment of CFT revealed a stabilization with a final mean value of 221 μm. In each of the scheduled visit sessions, the mean differences with respect to the baseline did not turn out to be statistically significant.

Our study demonstrates that at 24 months of follow-up, the IVBI offers the greatest chance to restore the initial VA loss in comparison to PDT or LT in patients affected by juxtafoveal myopic CNV, with documented VA deterioration. However, considering the small sample of this study and the relative low frequency of JCNV secondary to PM, a multicentric clinical trial with a longer follow-up is necessary to validate our results.

References

1 Hotchkiss ML, Fine SL: Pathologic myopia and choroidal neovascularization. Am J Ophthalmol 1981;91:177–183.
2 Curtin BJ: Basic science and clinical management; in Curtin BJ (ed): The Myopias. Philadelphia, Harper & Row, 1985, pp 237–245.
3 Tokoro T: Criteria for diagnosis of pathologic myopia; in Tokoro T (ed): Atlas of Posterior Fundus Changes in Pathologic Myopia. New York, Springer, 1998, pp 1–2.
4 Grossniklaus HE, Green WR: Pathologic findings in pathologic myopia. Retina 1992;12:127–133.
5 Avila MP, Weiter JJ, Jalkh AE, et al: Natural history of choroidal neovascularization in degenerative myopia. Ophthalmology 1984;91:1573–1581.
6 Grossniklaus HE, Gass JDM: Clinicopathologic correlations of surgically excised type 1 and type 2 submacular choroidal neovascular membranes. Am J Ophthalmol 1998;126:59–69.
7 Takeshi Y, Kyoko OM, Kenjiro Y, et al: Myopic choroidal neovascularization: a 10-year follow-up. Ophthalmology 2003;110:1297–1305.
8 Vongphanit J, Mitchell P, Wang JJ: Prevalence and progression of myopic retinopathy in an older population. Ophthalmology 2002;109:704–711.
9 Yoshida T, Ohno-Matsui K, Ohtake Y, et al: Long-term visual prognosis of choroidal neovascularization in high myopia. Ophthalmology 2002;109:712–719.
10 Yoshida T, Ohno-Matsui K, Yasazumi K, et al: Myopic choroidal neovascularization: a 10-year follow-up. Ophthalmology 2003;110:1297–1305.
11 Bottoni F, Tilanus M: The natural history of juxtafoveal and subfoveal choroidal neovascularization in high myopia. Int Ophthalmol 2001;24:249–255.
12 Hayashi K, Ohno-Matsui K, Yoshida T, Kobayashi K, Kojima A, Shimada N, Yasuzumi K, Futagami S, Tokoro T, Mochizuki M: Characteristics of patients with a favorable natural course of myopic choroidal neovascularization. Graefes Arch Clin Exp Ophthalmol 2005;243:13–19.
13 Brancato R, Menchini U, Pece A, et al: Dye laser photocoagulation of macular subretinal neovascularization in pathological myopia. A randomized study of three different wavelengths. Int Ophthalmol 1988;11:235–238.
14 Fardeau C, Soubrane G, Coscas G: Photocoagulation de néovaisseaux sous-rétinien compliquant la dégénérescence myopique. Bull Soc Ophtalmol Fr 1992; 3:239–242.
15 Soubrane G, Pisan J, Bornert P, Perrenoud F, Coscas G: Néovaisseaux sous-retiniens de la myopie dégénérative: résultats de la photocoagulation. Bull Soc Ophtalmol Fr 1986;86:269–272.
16 Secretan M, Kuhn D, Soubrane G, et al: Long-term visual outcome of choroidal neovascularization in pathologic myopia: natural history and laser treatment. Eur J Ophthalmol 1997;7:307–316.
17 Cohen SY, Bulik A, Dubois L, Quentel G: Photodynamic therapy for juxtafoveal choroidal neovascularization in myopic eyes. Am J Ophthalmol 2003; 136:371–374.
18 Lam DS, Liu DT, Fan DS, et al: Photodynamic therapy with verteporfin for juxtafoveal choroidal neovascularization secondary to pathologic myopia: one-year results of a prospective series. Eye 2005; 19:834–840.
19 Verteporfin in Photodynamic Therapy (VIP) Study Group: Photodynamic therapy of subfoveal choroidal neovascularization in pathologic myopia with verteporfin: one-year results of a randomized clinical trial - VIP report No. 1. Ophthalmology 2001; 108:841–852.
20 Blinder KJ, Blumenkranz MS, Bressler NM, et al: Verteporfin therapy of subfoveal choroidal neovascularization in pathologic myopia: two-year results of a randomized clinical trial – VIP report No. 3. Ophthalmology 2003;110:667–673.
21 Kobayashi H, Kobayashi K: Radiotherapy for subfoveal neovascularization associated with pathological myopia: a pilot study. Br J Ophthalmol 2000;84: 761–766.

22 Ruiz-Moreno JM, de la Vega C: Surgical removal of subfoveal choroidal neovascularization in highly myopic patients. Br J Ophthalmol 2001;85:1041–1043.

23 Hamelin N, Glacet-Bernard A, Brindeau C, et al: Surgical treatment of subfoveal neovascularization in myopia: macular translocation versus surgical removal. Am J Ophthalmol 2002;133:530–536.

24 Ferrara N, Gerber HP, LeCouter J: The biology of VEGF and its receptors. Nat Med 2003;9:669–676.

25 Sakaguchi H, Ikuno Y, Kamei M, et al: Intravitreal injection of bevacizumab for choroidal neovascularisation associated with pathological myopia. Br J Ophthalmol 2007;91:161–165.

26 Mandal S, Venkatesh P, Sampangi R, et al: Intravitreal bevacizumab (avastin) as primary treatment for myopic choroidal neovascularization. Eur J Ophthalmol 2007;17:620–626.

27 Rensch F, Spandau UH, Schlichtenbrede F, et al: Intravitreal bevacizumab for myopic choroidal neovascularization. Ophthalmic Surg Lasers Imaging 2008;39:182–185.

28 Gharbiya M, Allievi F, Mazzeo L, Gabrieli CB: Intravitreal bevacizumab treatment for choroidal neovascularization in pathologic myopia: 12-month results. Am J Ophthalmol 2009;147:84–93.

29 Wu PC, Chen YJ: Intravitreal injection of bevacizumab for myopic choroidal neovascularization: one-year follow-up. Eye 2009;23:356–361.

30 Ikuno Y, Sayanagi K, Soga K, et al: Intravitreal bevacizumab for choroidal neovascularization attributable to pathological myopia: one-year results. Am J Ophthalmol 2009;147:94–100.

31 Ruiz-Moreno JM, Montero JA, Gomez-Ulla F, Ares S: Intravitreal bevacizumab to treat subfoveal choroidal neovascularisation in highly myopic eyes: one-year outcome. Br J Ophthalmol 2009;93:448–451.

32 Chan WM, Lai TY, Chan KP, et al: Intravitreal bevacizumab (avastin) for myopic choroidal neovascularisation: one-year results of a prospective pilot study. Br J Ophthalmol 2009;93:150.

33 Hayashi K, Ohno-Matsui K, Shimada N, et al: Intravitreal bevacizumab on myopic choroidal neovascularization that was refractory to or had recurred after photodynamic therapy. Graefes Arch Clin Exp Ophthalmol 2009;247:609–618.

34 Ruiz-Moreno JM, Gomez-Ulla F, Montero JA, et al: Intravitreous bevacizumab to treat subfoveal choroidal neovascularization in highly myopic eyes: short-term results. Eye 2009;23:334–348.

35 Lai TY, Chan WM, Liu DT, Lam DS: Intravitreal ranibizumab for the primary treatment of choroidal neovascularization secondary to pathologic myopia. Retina 2009;29:750–756.

36 Silva RM, Ruiz-Moreno JM, Nascimento J, et al: Short-term efficacy and safety of intravitreal ranibizumab for myopic choroidal neovascularization. Retina 2008;28:1117–1123.

37 Arias L, Planas L, Prades S, et al: Intravitreal bevacizumab (avastin) for choroidal neovascularisation secondary to pathologic myopia: six-month results. Br J Ophthalmol 2008;92:1035–1039.

38 Axer-Siegel L, Ehrlich R, Weimberger D, et al: Photodynamic therapy of subfoveal choroidal neovascularization in high myopia in a clinical setting: visual outcome in relation to age at treatment. Am J Ophthalmol 2004;138:602–607.

Francesco Bandello, MD, FEBO
Professor and Chairman, Department of Ophthalmology
University Vita-Salute Scientific Institute, San Raffaele
Via Olgettina, 60, IT–20132 Milan (Italy)
Tel. +39 02 26432648, Fax +39 02 26483643, E-Mail francesco.bandello@hsr.it

Bandello F, Battaglia Parodi M (eds): Anti-VEGF.
Dev Ophthalmol. Basel, Karger, 2010, vol 46, pp 84–95

Antivascular Endothelial Growth Factors for Inflammatory Chorioretinal Disorders

Maurizio Battaglia Parodi[a] · Pierluigi Iacono[b] · Frank D. Verbraak[c] · Francesco Bandello[a]

[a]Department of Ophthalmology, University Vita-Salute, Scientific Institute San Raffaele, Milan; [b]Fondazione G.B. Bietti per l'Oftalmologia, Istituto di Ricovero e Cura a Carattere Scientifico, Rome, Italy, and [c]Academic Medical Center, Department of Ophthalmology, Amsterdam, The Netherlands

Abstract

Macular edema (ME) and choroidal neovascularization (CNV) can complicate the course of several inflammatory chorioretinal diseases, leading to a severe visual function impairment. The most frequently involved clinical entities include for example multifocal choroiditis, presumed ocular histoplasmosis syndrome, Beçhet's disease, multiple evanescent white dot syndrome, birdshot chorioretinopathy, acute multifocal posterior placoid pigment epitheliopathy, serpiginous choroiditis, and persistent placoid maculopathy. Results that have reported on antivascular endothelial growth factor (anti-VEGF) treatment in uveitic patients with CNV or ME have demonstrated positive results in many cases. However, bearing in mind that it has been proven impossible to perform randomized clinical trials with anti-VEGF in uveitic patients with CNV or ME, further studies with longer follow-ups are necessary to assess the value of this therapeutic approach.

Macular edema (ME) and choroidal neovascularization (CNV) can complicate the course of several inflammatory chorioretinal diseases, leading to a severe visual function impairment. ME can be ascribed to the dysfunction of or the damage to either the inner or the outer blood-retinal barrier. CNV development can be related to a number of features, comprising retinal pigment epithelium (RPE) damage and interruption of Bruch's membrane. Many cytokines and other molecules involved in the inflammatory process are also implicated in the pathogenetic mechanisms leading to a profound alteration of vascular permeability and angiogenesis.

Systemic or topical treatments aiming at reducing the inflammatory reaction often do not fully control ME and CNV development, and do not allow a recovery of the visual function. The recent advent of intravitreal antivascular endothelial growth factor (anti-VEGF) therapy has opened new perspectives for the treatment of ME and

CNV of inflammatory origin. Although the evidence supporting the use of anti-VEGF therapy in inflammatory chorioretinal diseases is not based on controlled trials, the positive results of a multitude of case series have demonstrated its value. These findings all support the beneficial effects of anti-VEGF molecules in the treatment of exudative complications of inflammatory chorioretinal disorders.

Inflammatory chorioretinal diseases comprise a heterogenous group of disorders. Some of these diseases are especially prone to the development of CNV, like multifocal choroiditis, presumed ocular histoplasmosis syndrome, Beçhet's disease, multiple evanescent white dot syndrome, birdshot chorioretinopathy, acute multifocal posterior placoid pigment epitheliopathy, serpiginous choroiditis, and persistent placoid maculopathy. Anti-VEGF therapy has been advocated for these diseases to successfully control CNV.

Most inflammatory chorioretinal diseases can lead to persistent uveitic cystoid macular edema (CME). Especially intermediate uveitis is known for this complication. Anti-VEGF therapy has been used to treat uveitic CME, and has shown promising results.

Multifocal Choroiditis and Punctate Inner Choriodopathy

Initially described by Nozik and Dorsch [1], multifocal choroiditis (MC) is a chronic inflammatory disease occurring most frequently in young, myopic, female subjects. Involvement of the anterior segment is detectable in about 50% of cases, whereas the posterior segment is invariably affected [1–10]. Typical features of the disorder are multiple punched-out chorioretinal lesions at the posterior pole and mid-periphery associated with vitritis. The visual prognosis in patients affected by MC is generally good, except for cases presenting macular involvement. A marked reduction in visual acuity (VA) is related to a number of complications, including CME, foveal scarring, epireretinal membrane, or CNV [1–10]. More specifically CNV has been reported as the most common cause of visual loss in MC, occurring in 27–32% of the cases [1–10].

Currently, there are no evidence-based guidelines for therapy of CNV secondary to MC. Some studies have described the beneficial effects of corticosteroid and immunosuppressant treatment, conventional laser treatment of extrafoveal CNV, and photodynamic therapy (PDT), and surgical excision for the management of sub- and juxtafoveal CNV [11–18].

Corticosteroid and immunosuppressant therapy have been reported to be beneficial in controlling the inflammation related to MC, but the efficacy in stabilizing the visual function in eyes with subfoveal CNV is still controversial [5, 8, 11–14]. Surgical CNV excision seems to offer good results, even though results are burdened with complications related to surgery, and a high recurrence rate [15, 16]. Small uncontrolled case series have reported that PDT can stabilize the visual function in eyes with sub- or juxtafoveal CNV, however without achieving a significant VA improvement [17–19].

Promising results have been reported with the use of intravitreal bevacizumab [20–22]. In particular, a retrospective study of the effect of bevacizumab administered for CNV not related to age-related macular degeneration also included 12 eyes affected by MC. The results were encouraging, even though a specific analysis is not allowed because only the cumulative results have been published [21]. More recently, Fine et al. [22] have reported on bevacizumab and ranibizumab intravitreal injections in 6 eyes affected by CNV secondary to MC. At the end of the available follow-up (mean follow-up 42 weeks, range 25–69 weeks), 5 eyes showed an improvement of the visual function with a final VA values better than 20/30 and reduced activity of CNV lesion. Only 1 patient experienced a reduction of visual function to 20/400 due to a subfoveal rip of the RPE. Anti-VEGF treatment will also inhibit the proinflammatory effects of VEGF present in these eyes.

The role of VEGF in the pathogenesis of CNV secondary to MC is supported by a recent study by Shimada et al. [23] who demonstrated that VEGF overexpression is detectable in samples of active CNV obtained after surgical excision. The pathology of excised neovascularizations did not differ between cases of MC or punctuate inner choroidopathy. An early neovascular 'bridging' between originally separated inflammatory and/or neovascular foci may bring about a severe VA loss after intravitreal bevacizumab therapy, however this is a process that can occur independent of any treatment, and the relation with the injection remains unclear [24].

Our experience refers to a prospective interventional case series including 10 eyes of 10 patients with MC-related subfoveal CNV, who underwent intravitreal bevacizumab injection, starting with three monthly injections, followed by retreatment as needed, with decisions to retreat based on loss of VA of more than 5 letters, and/or signs of active leakage on optical coherence tomography (OCT), over a 12-month follow-up. Mean best corrected VA (BCVA) and mean foveal thickness (FT) at the baseline were 0.58 logMAR (±0.48 SD) and 290 μm (±92 μm SD), respectively. At the 3-month examination, mean BCVA improved to 0.42 ± 0.48 and mean FT decreased to 268 ± 172 μm SD, whereas at the 12-month examination, mean BCVA was 0.40 ± 0.49 and mean FT was 255 ± 163 μm. Moreover, at the 12-month examination, 83% of patients showed a final VA better than 20/50, and overall, 9 out of 12 treated eyes (75%) showed at least one line of BCVA improvement, whereas 3 eyes (25%) revealed one line of worsening. The mean number of administered injections was 3.8, ranging from 3 to 7.

All the studies regarding the treatment of MC-related CNV have important limitations, especially the small number of patients and the absence of a control group. MC is a rare condition which makes the planning of a randomized clinical trial difficult. However, the reported improvement in VA in patients treated with anti-VEGF injections seems promising enough to consider this treatment in patients with multifocal choroiditis and a juxta- or subfoveal CNV.

Ocular Histoplasmosis Syndrome

Ocular histoplasmosis syndrome (OHS) is determined by the systemic infection of *Histoplasma capsulatum* and occurs in areas where *H. capsulatum* is endemic. Outside these endemic areas a similar ocular syndrome is recognized without any evidence of *H. capsulatum* and has been called ocular histoplasmosis. OHS is characterized by small, round, mid-peripheral chorioretinal lesions and peripapillary atrophy [25]. CNV is a well-known complication of OHS, which may lead to metamorphopsia and severe VA loss.

Fluorescein angiography evaluation of OHS reveals the presence of initially hypofluorescent spots which show staining in the late phases. Indocyanine green angiography unveils both hyper- and hypofluorescent spots, which often are not detectable on clinical examination. CNV secondary to OHS typically occurs during the second to fifth decade of life and shows a rapid course [25, 26]. Up to 75% of patients with CNV secondary to OHS experience a decline in vision to 20/200 or worse over the course of a 2- to 3-year period [27, 28]. Possible treatment options for CNV associated with OHS include laser photocoagulation, extrafoveal CNV, systemic and intravitreal corticosteroids, PDT, and surgical removal or macular displacement surgery, but all these treatment modalities have turned out to provide limited results regarding preservation of VA, sometimes with severe complications, and have shown a high recurrence rate [29–36].

In the absence of a beneficial treatment for OHS-related CNV, some authors have administered intravitreal anti-VEGF drugs. Positive functional and anatomical outcomes have been described in a single case report, with VA improvement from 20/200 to 20/60 over a 1-year follow-up and a single intravitreal injection of bevacizumab [37].

A retrospective interventional case series of 28 patients presenting either juxta- or subfoveal CNV related to OHS has demonstrated that intravitreal bevacizumab leads to a VA improvement in 71% eyes and a stabilization in 14% of cases over an average follow-up of 22 weeks [38]. Interestingly, all the patients presenting treatment-naive CNV stabilized or improved, in contrast to eyes previously treated with PDT or that received a combined treatment. This finding is consistent with published data about treatment results of CNV in AMD patients, where PDT-naive patients responded better [39].

Again a randomized controlled trial with a large number of patients would be needed to prove the effectiveness, safety, and long-term results of this therapy, but the results of the reported case series seems promising enough to consider this treatment in patients with OHS and a juxta- or subfoveal CNV.

Behçet's Disease

Behçet's disease is a complex systemic inflammatory disease with a severe inflammatory ocular involvement as one of the major manifestations of the disease. More specifically, the macula becomes involved with the development of CME, and, very seldom, a subfoveal CNV. A recent article has shown that intravitreal bevacizumab injection can be beneficial in the treatment of CME secondary to ocular Behçet's disease. In this investigation, 12 eyes of 11 patients underwent an intravitreal injection of bevacizumab. The results were encouraging showing a BCVA improvement in 7 eyes (58%), although the FT and macular volume, measured with OCT, did not reveal a statistically significant difference with respect to the baseline values [40]. More studies are needed to assess the value of the anti-VEGF approach in the therapy of ME secondary to Behçet's disease.

Multiple Evanescent White Dot Syndrome

Multiple evanescent white dot syndrome (MEWDS), originally described by Jampol et al. [41], is an acute, usually unilateral chorioretinopathy that occurs mostly in young subjects. Affected patients report blurred vision, photopsia, or visual field defects. MEWDS is clinically characterized by multiple yellow or white spots throughout the posterior pole and the peripheral retina, and punctated lesions surrounding the fovea.

Fluorescein angiography shows hyperfluorescence of the yellow spots, with diffuse or patchy staining at the RPE level and possible optic disc staining during the late phases. Early indocyanine green angiography demonstrates a pattern of hypofluorescent spots which are more apparent and more numerous with respect to the simple biomicroscopic examination. Such lesions varied in size from 50 to 500 μm in diameter [42]. Full-field and multifocal electroretinograms disclose dysfunction at the photoreceptors level [43, 44]. A typical OCT finding is the disruption of the photoreceptor inner/outer segment junction line which can recover along with the resolution of the disease [45]. The prognosis is generally good with complete spontaneous resolution of the inflammation within 6 months [45]. Nevertheless, subsequent recurrence, bilateral involvement or CNV development have been reported [46].

Intravitreal anti-VEGF has been employed to treat CNV which may complicate the course of the disease. In particular, a single case presenting peripapillary CNV and central subretinal fluid was treated by means of a single intravitreal injection of ranibizumab, achieving a positive functional and anatomical outcome. BCVA improved from 20/40 to 20/20, the CNV completely regressed, and the MEWDS findings disappeared over a follow-up of 6 months [47].

Birdshot Chorioretinopathy

The clinical manifestation of birdshot chorioretinopathy (BCR) is characterized by a posterior segment involvement with vitritis, 'birdshot' appearance of scattered, subretinal spots located anywhere in the fundus, but more frequently nasal to the optic disc and in the inferior retina. The lesions are oval, non-pigmented, creamy yellow, and flat with indistinct margins [48–51]. Macular and optic disc edema, CNV, and vasculitis may complicate the clinical picture [48–51]. HLA-A29 testing is very useful to confirm the diagnosis [52].

Electroretinography may reveal a decreased b-wave amplitude and delayed implicit time, especially in scotopic condition [51]. Fluorescein angiography shows early hypofluorescence and late hyperfluorescence of the spots. The optic disc usually reveals a dye leakage or staining, indicating the inflammatory involvement. On indocyanine green angiography the spots are hypofluorescent throughout the course of the examination. Many more spots are visible on indocyanine green angiography than with either biomicroscopy or fluorescein angiography. Very rarely, BCR may be complicated by the occurrence of a foveal CNV.

A case of BCR complicated by subfoveal CNV has been reported in an interventional case series including CNV forms other than AMD. The patient had previously received an intravitreous injection of triamcinolone acetonide without beneficial response and was retreated with intravitreal bevacizumab achieving a regression of the CNV [21]. An additional case with positive response to intravitreal bevacizumab was included in another case series [53].

BRC is more frequently complicated by chronic diffuse CME that can extend over the whole posterior pole. Interestingly, in a case of BRC presenting with CME, an improvement of BCVA in association with a reduction of the retinal thickness was reported after a single intravitreal injection of bevacizumab [54]. Experience with anti-VEGF in this disease is limited and needs further investigation.

Acute Multifocal Posterior Placoid Pigment Epitheliopathy

Acute multifocal posterior placoid pigment epitheliopathy (AMPPPE) is an acute self-limiting chorioretinal inflammatory disorder characterized by the development of multifocal, yellow-white, flat, placoid lesions at the level of the RPE at the posterior pole and at the mid-peripheral fundus [55]. The disease usually presents with an acute loss of vision. During the first weeks the expansion of the placoid lesions can occur, while new lesions can appear in formerly unaffected areas. This process continues for a few months with the development of new lesions and the healing of the older ones. Eventually all the lesions resolve, leading to the typical clinical aspect characterized by mottling, atrophy, and hyperpigmentation of the RPE, generally associated with a good functional recovery. The fluorescein angiograms during the acute phases show early hypofluorescence followed by staining of the lesions in the later phases. The indocyanine green angiograms reveal a choroidal hypofluorescence during the whole examination. Generally, AMPPPE has a good long-term prognosis for VA, although most patients have residual symptoms and paracentral scotomas [56]. Seldom, AMPPPE can lead to a severe loss of vision due to atrophic macular changes, subretinal fibrosis and CNV [57–60]. More specifically, CNV is a very rare complication of AMPPPE [61, 62]. As a consequence, no proven treatment is currently available for this complication. A single case report has recently described a 14-year-old girl who developed CNV as a complication of AMPPPE. The patient was effectively treated with a single intravitreal ranibizumab injection. BCVA improved from 20/40 to 20/20 through a follow-up of 12 months along with stabilization of the CNV and progressive reduction of subretinal fluid on OCT [63].

Serpiginous Choroiditis

Serpiginous choroiditis (SC) is a rare, progressive, chronically recurring inflammatory disorder. SC is usually bilateral, with onset between the ages of 30 and 70 years, and no race or sex predilection [64–67]. SC is characterized by the occurrence of grayish-yellow lesions at the RPE level, most frequently located close to the optic disc with peripapillary lesions and fingerlike projections extending outward. In rare cases the disease takes place in the macula, or in other retinal areas, without peripapillary involvement [67]. The active lesions last from weeks to months and then there is a spontaneous resolution with pigment loss or clumping and retinochoroidal atrophy [68]. Patients affected by SC have typically recurrences at intervals varying from weeks to years, with extension to the periphery. About one third of patients reveal an inflammatory reaction in the posterior and the anterior segment [66, 69].

Occasionally, findings of SC may be associated with other manifestations, including retinal vasculitis, papillitis, vitritis, branch retinal vein occlusion, serous neurosensory detachment, RPE detachment, and optic disc neovascularization [70–72]. CNV occurs in up to 35% of cases of SC and may be seen at the time of active choroiditis or in between episodes [72–75]. The treatment of the CNV secondary to SC is still debated, but a recent case report has described a favorable outcome after treatment with intravitreal injection of ranibizumab [76]. Other studies are necessary to validate the clinical relevance of this therapy.

Persistent Placoid Maculopathy

Persistent placoid maculopathy (PPM) is a new clinical entity characterized by bilateral symmetric macular involvement characterized by a whitish plaque-like lesion at the level of the RPE centered around the fovea, which is often complicated by CNV development with disciform evolution [77, 78]. Owing to the rarity of this complication, currently there is no proven treatment able to manage PPM-related CNV. Corticosteroids have been tried in a previous report, without halting the progression toward CNV development and disciform scarring [77, 78].

We have diagnosed and treated a 60-year-old man affected by PPM and bilateral CNV [79]. At presentation, BCVA was 20/800 in the right eye, due to an old fibrovascular scar as a result of the natural evolution of a subfoveal CNV, and 20/32 in the left eye, which hosted a juxtafoveal CNV. The patient was treated with intravitreal injection of 1.25 mg bevacizumab in the left eye. One week later, BCVA in the treated eye was 20/25 and a partial resolution of the subretinal fluid on OCT could be noticed. At the 30-day examination, BCVA was still 20/25, with persistence of minimal intraretinal fluid, and some dye leakage on fluorescein angiography. A second treatment was provided and 1 week later, BCVA improved to 20/20 with complete resolution of fluid on OCT. Fluorescein angiography revealed the absence of dye leakage. The patient has been followed up monthly for 18 months, without registering any further change on OCT and angiography.

Uveitic Cystoid Macular Edema

CME is the most common cause of significant visual loss in patients affected by intraocular inflammation [80]. The actual incidence of uveitic CME differs according to the underlying etiology and inflammation site. In particular, CME has been registered in about 30% of HLA-B27-positive patients with anterior uveitis, as compared with 8% of HLA-B27-negative patients [81, 82]. CME is associated more commonly with more posterior locations of uveitis (intermediate, posterior, and panuveitis) [83]. The pathogenesis of uveitic CME is not completely understood and may result from dysfunction of and/or damage to either the inner or the outer blood-retinal barrier. Many inflammatory cytokines and other molecules such as arachidonic acid have been implicated in the etiology of this common complication, and it is probable that a combination of different factors concur to the development of this condition [84]. Untreated uveitic CME tends to cause progressive visual loss because of a progressive photoreceptor damage. Medical treatment includes several approaches, such as topical and systemic non-steroidal anti-inflammatory drugs, corticosteroids (topical, systemic, transseptal, or intravitreal), systemic carbonic anhydrase inhibitors, and octreotide [85]. The difficulties in obtaining a favorable functional outcome together with the resistance to the treatment modalities have led several authors to search for new therapies. A recent investigation has taken into consideration 13 patients with CME secondary to different uveitic forms, causing significant visual impairment, who were resistant to medical therapy including not only initial use of topical and/or systemic anti-inflammatory drugs, but also to intravitreal injections of triamcinolone acetonide in the majority of cases [54]. The use of intravitreal bevacizumab achieved encouraging results, with significant improvement in vision and central retinal thickness in patients with this type of recalcitrant CME. Survival analysis showed that the probability of any improvement in VA increased progressively starting at 6 weeks and reached 81% at 14 weeks. These preliminary data suggest that intravitreal bevacizumab may be a beneficial choice for the treatment of recalcitrant uveitic CME, and more definitive studies into this matter are warranted.

Conclusions

Anti-VEGF treatment in uveitic patients has been provided for two reasons: the development of CNV and persistent, treatment-resistant ME. Choroidal neovascularizations in uveitic patients are frequently seen in some diseases entities like MC, but are a more rare complication in others. In the development of CNV in uveitic patients, more so than in AMD patients, inflammations play a pivotal role. Anti-inflammatory drugs, locally or systemically given, can be effective in the treatment of CNV in many cases, but the response may be too slow, leaving the eye permanently damaged, with loss of VA, which can be profound in patients with involvement of the fovea. Anti-VEGF could be a solution for this problem and could be especially helpful in preventing this permanent loss of vision in the acute phase of diseases. This approach is interesting because it directly acts on the pathogenetic mechanisms of the CNV development, eliminating the inflammatory rebound typical of other treatment modalities, such as laser photocoagulation or PDT.

In some uveitic diseases, like Beçhet's disease, BCR, SC, adequate immune suppression, most of the time requiring systemic corticosteroids in combination with other immune suppressors like methotrexate, azathioprine or mycophenolate, cyclosporine, is mandatory in addition to intraocular anti-VEGF. While in others, with less inflammation, like OHS or multifocal choroiditis, anti-VEGF could probably be sufficient to treat the CNV adequately. The role of treatment with anti-VEGF in CME is more controversial and should probably be reserved for those cases that are unresponsive to other anti-inflammatory treatments, although here again the anti-inflammatory effect of anti-VEGF will be beneficial, albeit probably only for a relatively short time.

Results reported on the anti-VEGF treatment in uveitic patients with CNV or ME have demonstrated positive results. However, as always, it has been proven impossible to perform randomized clinical trials with anti-VEGF in uveitic patients with CNV or ME, and for the time being we will have to base our treatment decisions not on evidence-based protocols, but on case series, the experience of others, and by one's own expertise and common sense.

References

1 Nozik RA, Dorsch W: A new chorioretinopathy associated with anterior uveitis. Am J Ophthalmol 1973;76:758–762.

2 Tatar O, Yoeruek E, Szurman P, et al: Effect of bevacizumab on inflammation and proliferation in human choroidal neovascularization. Arch Ophthalmol 2008;126:782–790.

3 Dryer RF, Gass JDM: Multifocal choroiditis and panuveitis. A syndrome that mimics ocular histoplasmosis. Arch Ophthalmol 1984;102:1776–1784.

4 Deutsch TA, Tessler HH: Inflammatory pseudohistoplasmosis. Ann Ophthalmol 1985;17:451–465.

5 Cantrill HL, Folk JC: Multifocal choroiditis associated with progressive subretinal fibrosis. Am J Ophthalmol 1986;101:170–180.

6 Morgan CM, Schatz H: Recurrent multifocal choroiditis. Ophthalmology 1986;93:1138–1147.

7 Lardenoye CW, Van der Lelij A, de Loos WS, et al: Peripheral multifocal chorioretinitis: a distinct clinical entity? Ophthalmology 1997;104:1820–1826.

8 Jampol LM, Wiredu A: MEWDS, MFC, PIC, AMN, AIBSE, and AZOOR: one disease or many? Retina 1995;15:373–378.

9 Brown J, Folk JC, Reddy CV, Kimura AE: Visual prognosis of multifocal choroiditis, punctate inner choroidopathy, and the diffuse subretinal fibrosis syndrome. Ophthalmology 1996;103:1100–1105.

10 Slakter JS, Giovannini A, Yannuzzi LA, et al: Indocyanine green angiography of multifocal choroiditis. Ophthalmology 1997;104:1813–1819.

11 Michel SS, Ekong A, Baltatzis S, Foster S: Multifocal choroiditis and panuveitis: immunomodulatory therapy. Ophthalmology 2002;109:378–383.

12 Flaxel CJ, Owens SL, Mulholland B, et al: The use of corticosteroids for choroidal neovascularisation in young patients. Eye 1998;12:266–272.

13 Nussenblatt RB, Coleman H, Jirawuthiworavong G, et al: The treatment of multifocal choroiditis associated choroidal neovascularization with sirolimus (rapamycin). Acta Ophthalmol Scand 2007;85:230–231.

14 Michel SS, Ekong A, Baltatzis S, Foster CS: Multifocal choroiditis and panuveitis: immunomodulatory therapy. Ophthalmology 2002;109:378–383.

15 Olsen TW, Capone A, Sternberg P, et al: Subfoveal choroidal neovascularization in punctate inner choroidopathy. Surgical management and pathologic findings. Ophthalmology 1996;103:2061–2069.

16 Thomas MA, Dickinson JD, Melberg NS, et al: Visual results after surgical removal of subfoveal choroidal neovascular membranes. Ophthalmology 1994;101:1384–1396.

17 Spaide RF, Freund KB, Slakter J, et al: Treatment of subfoveal choroidal neovascularization associated with multifocal choroiditis and panuveitis with photodynamic therapy. Retina 2002;22:545–549.

18 Parodi MB, Di Crecchio L, Lanzetta P, et al: Photodynamic therapy with verteporfin for subfoveal choroidal neovascularization associated with multifocal choroiditis. Am J Ophthalmol 2004;138:263–269.

19 Parodi MB, Iacono P, Spasse S, Ravalico G: Photodynamic therapy for juxtafoveal choroidal neovascularization associated with multifocal choroiditis. Am J Ophthalmol 2006;141:23–26.

20 Chan WM, Lai TY, Liu DT, Lam DS: Intravitreal bevacizumab (Avastin) for choroidal neovascularization secondary to central serous chorioretinopathy, secondary to punctate inner choroidopathy, or of idiopathic origin. Am J Ophthalmol 2007;143:977–983.

21 Chang LK, Spaide RF, Brue C, et al: Bevacizumab treatment for subfoveal choroidal neovascularization from causes other than age-related macular degeneration. Arch Ophthalmol 2008;126:941–945.

22 Fine HF, Zhitomirsky IB, Freund KB, et al: Bevacizumab (Avastin) and ranibizumab (Lucentis) for choroidal neovascularization in multifocal choroiditis. Retina 2009;29:8–12.

23 Shimada H, Yuzawa M, Hirose T, et al: Pathological findings of multifocal choroiditis with panuveitis and punctate inner choroidopathy. Jpn J Ophthalmol 2008;52:282–288.

24 Reche-Frutos J, Calvo-Gonzalez C, Donate-Lopez J, Garcia-Feijoo J: Early neovascular bridging of choroidal neovascularization after ranibizumab treatment. Graefes Arch Clin Exp Ophthalmol 2009;247:1427–1430.

25 Prasad AG, Van Gelder RN: Presumed ocular histoplasmosis syndrome. Curr Opin Ophthalmol 2005;16:364–368.

26 Brown DM, Weingeist TA, Smith RE: Histoplasmosis; in Pepose JS, Holland GN, Wilhelmus KR (eds): Ocular Infection and Immunity. St Louis, Mosby, 1996, pp 1252–1261.

27 Kleiner RC, Ratner CM, Enger C, Fine SL: Subfoveal neovascularization in the ocular histoplasmosis syndrome: a natural history study. Retina 1988;8:225–229.

28 Ciulla TA, Piper HC, Xiao M, Wheat LJ: Presumed ocular histoplasmosis syndrome: update on epidemiology, pathogenesis, and photodynamic, antiangiogenic, and surgical therapies. Curr Opin Opthalmol 2001;12:442–449.

29 Olk JR, Burgess DB, McCormick PA: Subfoveal and juxtafoveal subretinal neovascularization in the presumed ocular histoplasmosis syndrome: visual prognosis. Ophthalmology 1984;91:1592–1602.

30 Macular Photocoagulation Study Group: Krypton laser photocoagulation for neovascular lesions of ocular histoplasmosis: results of a randomized clinical trial. Arch Ophthalmol 1987;105:1499–1507.

31 Martidis A, Miller DG, Ciulla TA, Danis RP, Moorthy RS: Corticosteroids as an antiangiogenic agent for histoplasmosis-related subfoveal choroidal neovascularization. J Ocul Pharmacol Ther 1999;15:425–428.

32 Rechtman E, Allen VD, Danis RP, et al, Intravitreal triamcinolone for choroidal neovascularization in ocular histoplasmosis syndrome. Am J Ophthalmol 2003;136:739–741.

33 Breger AS, Conway M, del Priore LV, et al: Submacular surgery for subfoveal choroidal neovascular membranes in patients with presumed ocular histoplasmosis. Arch Ophthalmol 1997;115:991–996.

34 Submacular Surgery Trials Research Group: Surgical removal vs. observation for subfoveal choroidal neovascularization, either associated with the ocular histoplasmosis syndrome or idiopathic. I. Ophthalmic findings from a randomized clinical trial: Submacular Surgery Trials (SST) Group H Trial: SST Report No 9. Arch Ophthalmol 2004;122:1597–1611.

35 Verteporfin in Ocular Histoplasmosis (VOH) Study Group: Photodynamic therapy of subfoveal choroidal neovascularization with verteporfin in the ocular histoplasmosis syndrome: one-year results of an uncontrolled, prospective case series. Ophthalmology 2002;109:1499–1505.
36 Verteporfin in Ocular Histoplasmosis Study Group: Photodynamic therapy with verteporfin in ocular histoplasmosis: uncontrolled, open-label two-year study. Ophthalmology 2004;111:1725–1733.
37 Adán A, Navarro M, Casaroli-Marano RP, et al: Intravitreal bevacizumab as initial treatment for choroidal neovascularization associated with presumed ocular histoplasmosis syndrome. Graefes Arch Clin Exp Ophthalmol 2007;245:1873–1875.
38 Schadlu R, Blinder KJ, Shah GK, et al: Intravitreal bevacizumab for choroidal neovascularization in ocular histoplasmosis. Am J Ophthalmol 2008;145:875–878.
39 Yoganathan P, Deramo VA, Lai JC, et al: Visual improvement following intravitreal bevacizumab (Avastin) in exudative age-related macular degeneration. Retina 2006;26:994–998.
40 Mirshahi A, Namavari S, Djalilian A, et al: Intravitreal bevacizumab (Avastin) for the treatment of cystoid macular edema in Beçhet's disease. Ocular Immunol Inflamm 2009;17:59–64.
41 Jampol LM, Sieving PA, Pugh D, et al: Multiple evanescent white dot syndrome. I. Clinical findings. Arch Ophthalmol 1984;102:671–674.
42 Gross NE, Yannuzzi LA, Freund KB, et al: Multiple evanescent white dot syndrome. Arch Ophthalmol 2006;124:493–500.
43 Sieving PA, Fishman GA, Jampol LM, Pugh D: Multiple evanescent white dot syndrome. II. Electrophysiology of the photoreceptors during retinal pigment epithelium disease. Arch Ophthalmol 1984;102:675–679.
44 Feigl B, Haas A, El-Shabrawi Y: Multifocal ERG in multiple evanescent white dot syndrome. Graefes Arch Clin Exp Ophthalmol 2002;240:615–621.
45 Li D, Kishi S: Restored photoreceptor outer segment damage in multiple evanescent white dot syndrome. Ophthalmology 2009:116:762–770.
46 Wyhinny GJ, Jackson JL, Jampol JM: Subretinal neovascularization following multiple evanescent white dot syndrome. Arch Ophthalmol 1990;108:1384.
47 Rouvas AA, Ladas ID, Papakostas TD, et al: Intravitreal ranibizumab in a patient with choroidal neovascularization secondary to multiple evanescent white dot syndrome. Eur J Ophthalmol 2007;17:996–999.
48 Ryan SJ, Maumenee AE: Birdshot retinochoroidopathy. Am J Ophthalmol 1980;89:31–45.
49 Soubrane G, Bokobza R, Coscas G: Late developing lesions in birdshot retinochoroidopathy. Am J Ophthalmol 1990;109:204–210.
50 Brucker AJ, Deglin EA, Bene C, Hoffman ME: Subretinal choroidal neovascularization in birdshot retinochoroidopathy. Am J Ophthalmol 1985;99:40–44.
51 Fuerst DJ, Tessler HH, Fishman GA, et al: Birdshot retinochoroidopathy. Arch Ophthalmol 1984;102:214–219.
52 Nussenblatt RB, Mittal KK, Ryan SJ, et al: Birdshot retinochoroidopathy associated with HLA-A20 antigen and immune responsiveness to retinal S-antigen. Am J Ophthalmol 1982;94:147–158.
53 Nguyen QD, Shah SM, Hafiz G, et al: intravitreal bevacizumab causes regression of choroidal neovascularization secondary to diseases other than age-related macular degeneration. Am J Ophthalmol 2008;145:257–266.
54 Cordero Coma M, Sobrin L, Onal S, et al: Intravitreal bevacizumab for treatment of uveitic macular edema. Ophthalmology 2007;114:1574–1579.
55 Gass JDM: Acute posterior multifocal placoid pigment epitheliopathy. Arch Ophthalmol 1968;80:177–185.
56 Wolf MD, Alward WL, Folk JC: Long-term visual function in acute posterior multifocal placoid pigment epitheliopathy. Arch Ophthalmol 1991;109:800–803.
57 Isashiki M, Koide H, Yamashita T, Ohba N: Acute posterior multifocal placoid pigment epitheliopathy associated with diffuse retinal vasculitis and late haemorrhagic macular detachment. Br J Ophthalmol 1986;70:255–259.
58 Williams DF, Mieler WF: Long-term follow-up of acute multifocal posterior placoid pigment epitheliopathy. Br J Ophthalmol 1989;73:985–990.
59 Daniele S, Daniele C, Orcidi F, Tavano A: Progression of choroidal atrophy in acute posterior multifocal placoid pigment epitheliopathy. Ophthalmologica 1998;212:66–72.
60 Pagliarini S, Piguet B, Ffytche TJ, Bird AC: Foveal involvement and lack of visual recovery in APMPPE associated with uncommon features. Eye 1995;9:42–47.
61 Bowie EM, Sletten KR, Kayser DL, Folk JC: Acute posterior multifocal placoid pigment epitheliopathy and choroidal neovascularization. Retina 2005;25:362–364.
62 Espinasse-Berrod MA, Gotte D, Parent de Curzon H, Bayen MC, Campinchi R: A case of multiple epitheliopathy associated with subretinal neovascularizations. J Fr Ophtalmol 1988;11:191–194.

63 Mavrakanas N, Mendrinos E, Tabatabay C, Pournaras CJ: Intravitreal ranibizumab for choroidal neovascularization secondary to acute multifocal posterior placoid pigment epitheliopathy. Acta Ophthalmol 2010;88:e54–e55.
64 Schatz H, Maumenee AE, Patz A: Geographic helicoid peripapillary choroidopathy: clinical presentation and fluorescein angiographic findings. Trans Am Acad Ophthalmol Otolaryngol 1974;78:747–751.
65 Blumenkranz MS, Gass JDM, Clarkson JG: Atypical serpiginous choroiditis. Arch Ophthalmol 1982;100:1773–1778.
66 Laatikainen L, Erkkila H: Serpiginous choroiditis. Br J Ophthalmol 1974;58:777–783.
67 Mansour AM, Jampol LK, Packo HK, Hrisalamos NF: Macular serpiginous choroiditis. Retina 1988;8:125–129.
68 Chisholm IH, Gass JDM, Hutton WL: The late stages of serpiginous (geographic) choroiditis. Am J Ophthalmol 1976;82:343–348.
69 Masi RJ, O'Connor R, Kimura SJ: Anterior uveitis in geographic or serpiginous choroiditis. Am J Ophthalmol 1978;86:228–231.
70 Sahel JA, Weber M, Conlon MR, Albert DM: Pathology of the uveal tract; in Albert DM, Jakobiec FA (eds): Principles and Practices of Ophthalmology: Clinical Practice. Philadelphia. Saunders, 1994, vol 182, pp 2145–2179.
71 Wojno T, Meredith TA: Unusual findings in serpiginous choroiditis. Am J Ophthalmol 1982;94:650–653.
72 Laatikainen L, Erkkila H: Subretinal and disc neovascularization in serpiginous choroiditis. Br J Ophthalmol 1982;66:326–328.
73 Jampol JK, Orth D, Daily MJ, Rabb MF: Subretinal neovascularization with geographic (serpiginous) choroiditis. Am J Ophthalmol 1979;88:683–686.
74 Gass JDM: Serpiginous Choroiditis. Stereoscopic Atlas of Macular Diseases: Diagnosis and Treatment, ed 4. St Louis, Mosby, 1997, pp 158–165.
75 Christmas NH, Ok KT, Oh DM, Folk JC: Long-term follow-up of patients with serpiginous choroiditis. Retina 2002;22:550–556.
76 Song MH, Roh YJ: Intravitreal ranibizumab for choroidal neovascularisation in serpiginous choroiditis. Eye (Lond) 2009;23:1873–1875.
77 Golchet PR, Jampol LM, Wilson D, Yannuzzi LA, Ober M, Stroh E: Persistent placoid maculopathy. A new clinical entity. Trans Am Ophthalmol Soc 2006;104:108–120.
78 Golchet PR, Jampol LM, Wilson D, Yannuzzi LA, Ober M, Stroh E: Persistent placoid maculopathy. A new clinical entity. Ophthalmology 2007;114:1530–1540.
79 Parodi MB, Iacono P, Bandello F: Juxtafoveal choroidal neovascularization secondary to persistent placoid maculopathy treated with intravitreal bevacizumab. In press.
80 Rothova A, Suttorp-van Schulten MS, Frits Treffers W, Kijlstra A: Causes and frequency of blindness in patients with intraocular inflammatory disease. Br J Ophthalmol 1996;80:332–336.
81 Rosenbaum JT: Characterization of uveitis associated with spondyloarthritis. J Rheumatol 1989;16:792–796.
82 Bayen H, Bayen MC, De Curzon HP, et al: Involvement of the posterior eye segment in HLA-B27^{+} iridocyclitis: incidence; value of surgical treatment. J Fr Ophtalmol 1988;11:561–566.
83 Markomichelakis NN, Halkiadakis I, Pantelia E, et al: Patterns of macular edema in patients with uveitis: qualitative and quantitative assessment using optical coherence tomography. Ophthalmology 2004;111:946–953.
84 Guex-Crosier Y: The pathogenesis and clinical presentation of macular edema in inflammatory diseases. Doc Ophthalmol 1999;97:297–309.
85 Papadaki T, Zacharopoulos I, Iaccheri B, et al: Somatostatin for uveitic cystoid macular edema. Ocul Immunol Inflamm 2005;13:469–470.

Francesco Bandello, MD, FEBO
Professor and Chairman, Department of Ophthalmology
University Vita-Salute Scientific Institute, San Raffaele
Via Olgettina, 60, IT–20132 Milan (Italy)
Tel. +39 02 2643 2648, Fax +39 02 2648 3643, E-Mail francesco.bandello@hsr.it

Bandello F, Battaglia Parodi M (eds): Anti-VEGF.
Dev Ophthalmol. Basel, Karger, 2010, vol 46, pp 96–106

Antivascular Endothelial Growth Factor Treatment in Pseudoxanthoma Elasticum Patients

Frank D. Verbraak

Departments of Ophthalmology and Biomedical Engineering & Physics, Academic Medical Center, Amsterdam, The Netherlands

Abstract

The eye in patients with pseudoxanthoma elasticum, an autosomal recessive disease, shows several lesions, like peau d'orange, angioid streaks, comet lesions, and paired hyperpigmented smudges. The most devastating ocular complication is the development of choroidal neovascularizations (CNV). This exudative disease of the central retina leads to loss of visual acuity, and results of treatments in the past have been disappointing. From the present evidence it may be concluded that intravitreal anti-vascular endothelial growth factor (anti-VEGF) therapy with ranibizumab or bevacizumaab is beneficial for the treatment of CNV secondary to angioid streaks associated with PXE. Especially in the early stages of the disease, visual acuity can be maintained or even improved over a prolonged period of time, even with a low number of injections. Later in the course of the disease, when more widespread atrophic changes have occurred, the perspective is more bleak. Although there seem to be arguments to treat selected patients with a maintenance treatment of intravitreal injections once every 2 months, an as-needed regimen is the most used strategy. Patients need to be aware of the off-label nature of the treatment with anti-VEGF and also need to be informed about the possible increased risk of cardio-vascular and/or thromboembolic events, although at present no definite proof has been documented of this higher risk in patients with or without PXE treated with intravitreal anti-VEGF. Overall, based on the evidence available, intravitreal treatment with anti-VEGF seems to be the best choice at present to treat patients with CNV secondary to angioid streaks and PXE.

History and General Disease

Pseudoxanthoma elasticum (PXE) was already described at the end of the 19th century by dermatologists. The characteristic ocular angioid streaks were described slightly later, but it was only as late as 1929 that the association between the two abnormalities was realized by the Swedish ophthalmologist Groenblad and the dermatologist Strandberg. The PXE syndrome has since their description also been known as the Groenblad-Strandberg syndrome [1–3].

The skin lesions precede the other manifestations and are most often the reason a patient is diagnosed as being affected by PXE. Small, 1–5 mm, soft papules with a yellowish color present themselves in a reticular pattern, already at the age of 13, but are most often diagnosed the first time at the age of 22 years. They occur typically on the neck, axillae, groin, and the back of the knee. Plaques or redundant skin have also been described. Although the skin lesions are very characteristic, they are not pathognomonic for PXE, nor does the absence of skin changes exclude a diagnosis of PXE [3–6].

Cardiovascular complications due to generalized calcification of tissues and vessels are often seen. Hypertension (22.5%), atherosclerosis (25%), intermittent claudicatio (18%), gastrointestinal hemorrhage (13%), angina pectoris (19%), and early myocardial infarction all belong to the spectrum of these complications, and to a large extent determine the course of the disease [2–6].

The eye shows several lesions, like peau d'orange, angioid streaks, comet lesions, and paired hyperpigmented smudges. The most devastating ocular complication is the development of choroidal neovascularizations (CNV). This exudative disease of the central retina leads to loss of visual acuity (VA), and results of treatment have been disappointing. However, as in exudative age-related macular degeneration (AMD), the use of antivascular endothelial growth factor (anti-VEGF) intraocular injections with ranibizumab or bevacizumab have been proven to maintain or even improve VA in many of these patients.

Genetics of PXE

Initially, PXE was considered to be sporadic, but it is now known to be an autosomal recessive disease. Cases with pseudodominance with diseased family members in two generations have been described, but never families with three generations. The prevalence in the general population is between 1 in 25,000 to 1 in 100,000 live births [1]. For years the disease was assumed to be caused by abnormal elastic fibers, and mutations were expected in the genes coding for the synthesis of elastic fibers, like elastin, fibrillin, or microfibrillar-associated proteins and/or enzymes, but were never found. Positional cloning of a linked 16d13.1 region, found through linkage analysis to be involved in PXE, identified a small region of 500 kb, which included 5 genes. Direct sequencing detected that mutations in one of these genes, the ABCC6 gene, was the cause of PXE. Up till now, more than 200 mutations in the ABCC6 gene have been identified to be the cause of PXE [1–3, 6–9].

The ABCC6 gene encodes for an ATP-binding cassette transporter (ABC), which actively transports from the intra- to the extracellular space or into cell compartments. The protein encoded by the gene regulates the calcium concentration, and reduces the calcium phosphate precipitation outside the cells. Loss of function leads to dystrophic mineralization and fragmentation of elastic fibers, abnormalities of collagen fibers, and defects in the extracellular matrix [10].

Interestingly, certain vascular endothelial growth factor gene polymorphisms seem to be a prognostic factor for the manifestation of CNV in patients with PXE [11]. The most significant single nucleotide polymorphism associated with the development of CNV was c.-460C>T, with an odds ratio of 3.83 (95% CI 2.01–7.31, $p = 0.0003$). These findings suggest an involvement of VEGF in the development of PXE-associated ocular manifestations. This VEGF gene polymorphism could also be used as a prognostic marker, identifying patients at high risk for the development of CNV.

Ocular Signs and Symptoms of PXE

Fine yellow drusen-like pigment abnormalities temporal of the fovea, peau d'orange, are the first visible lesions in the eye of patients with PXE. These abnormalities are located at the level of the retinal pigment epithelium (RPE), and do not influence retinal function. No histological correlates have been identified for these changes. It is one of the typical lesions seen in PXE, but can be highly variable in expression. It can be seen in over 90% of PXE patients with the typical skin lesions [12–14].

Later in life the angioid streaks become visible, usually not before the age of 10 years [2, 12, 13]. They originate from the optic disc, sometimes even encircle the disk, and radiate towards the periphery in an irregular pattern, as brownish lines with a varying width. The prevalence of angioid streaks is as high as 99% 20 years following the diagnosis of PXE in patients [2, 12, 13]. Peau d'orange and angioid streaks are usually bilateral. The angioid streaks most often are easily recognized, but sometimes small angioid streaks are difficult to identify. On angiography, especially indocyanine green angiography, the angioid streaks are much more pronounced, and can more easily be identified [15, 16]. Once formed, the angioid streaks seem to remain stationary, although long-term studies have shown a slow increase in width and length over the years. Late in the course of the disease, angioid streaks become more atrophic, an atrophy that extends to the adjacent RPE and choriocapillaris, and can lead to large areas of atrophy in the center of the macula [12, 17].

In an autofluorescence study of patients with PXE, abnormalities were detected in the RPE-photoreceptor complex that were more widespread than expected from conventional fundus imaging [18]. Lobular or multilobular and diffuse areas of RPE atrophy could be found in 72% of the examined eyes. The extensive alteration of the RPE suggested an important role of pathologic RPE changes in the evolution of visual loss in PXE patients, also in the absence of neovascularizations. The RPE changes correlate with changes in Bruch's membrane that shows thickening and calcification over large areas. In addition, a pattern dystrophy-like alteration is also part of the spectrum of macular changes, seen in 10% of cases, and could also be associated with progressive vision loss.

In the mid-periphery, comet-like lesions have been found in PXE patients [2, 14, 19, 20]. These chorioretinal atrophic lesions present in 60% of patients show a localized

RPE and underlying choroid atrophy with a slightly depigmented tail pointing from the lesion towards the posterior pole, like a comet's tail. They seem to be pathognomonic for PXE. The lesions are generally small (around 125 μm) and located outside the fovea, and do not influence vision. Another asymptomatic ocular sign present in 50% of PXE patients is the presence of paired hyperpigmented smudges, like the wings of a predator bird, aligning an angioid streak [12]. A non-specific ocular finding, associated with angioid streaks, is the presence of optic disc drusen that can be present in up to 20% of patients [21].

Secondary hemorrhagic and exudative changes in the macula can be found in 73–86% of the cases [2, 13, 17, 22–24]. In contrast to the other manifestations of PXE, these lesions do lead to a profound loss of VA. Small traumata can cause severe bleeding and cause extensive subretinal hemorrhages, especially around angiod streaks. Patients should be made aware of this risk and avoid unnecessary traumata [24].

CNV's develop, which grow through the breaks in Bruch's membrane at the site of angioid streaks. In contrast to AMD a CNV in PXE develops at a much younger age. In many cases the first presentation is juxtafoveal, and not subfoveal as in AMD, however later on in the course of the disease, the recurrences will include the fovea. Many cases become bilateral within 1–2 years [2, 13, 22, 23, 25–28].

Treatment of CNV

The treatment of CNV associated with the angioid streaks seen in PXE before the use of anti-VEGF injections had only a very limited efficacy. Laser photocoagulation, transpupillary thermotherapy, selective indocyanine green-mediated photothrombosis of ingrowth site vessels, and rare cases of macular translocation have all been used in the past, and with these treatments stability of the lesions was the best result in some series, but most patients continued to lose their VA [29–34]. The best results were reported with photodynamic therapy (PDT), with or without additional intraocular injection with triamcinolone, but unfortunately, also PDT was not able to stop the progression of the development of CNV, and perhaps also due to the unwanted collateral damage inherent to this treatment, vision loss could not be stopped [35].

The success of anti-VEGF treatment of CNV in other diseases encouraged many ophthalmologists to treat patients with CNV due to angioid streaks off-label with either bevacizumab or ranibizumab. The rarity of the disease prevented large series to be studied, and most case series did have a relatively short follow-up [28, 36–43]. However, the results were very encouraging.

Two larger case series were reported and one of these also reported on the long-term outcomes, after a follow-up of more than 24 months [39, 42] (table 1). In these two series a total of 11 women and 14 men were treated with a mean age of 53 years (range 24–72). Mean follow-up was 8.6 months in the study by Finger et al. [39], patients 1–15, and 28.5 months in the study by Myung et al. [42], patients 16–24.

Table 1. Patients treated with bevacizumab

Patient No.	Gender	Age	Previous treatment	Best corrected VA		Follow-up, months	Injections, n
				baseline	final		
1	F	46		20/25	20/20	10	2
2	M	38		20/200	20/50	5	2
3	M	24		20/63	20/16	2	2
4	M	46	PDT	20/20	20/16	3	1
5	M	47		20/400	20/50	9	1
	M			20/100	20/50	14	1
6	M	60		20/40	20/32	4	3
7	F	44		20/63	20/800	3	1
8	M	50		20/160	20/160	11	1
9	F	61		20/200	20/80	6	2
10	M	72	PDT	20/40	20/32	19	1
11	F	66		20/2,000	20/125	12	2
12	F	65	PDT	20/50	20/80	4	1
13	M	57		20/250	20/400	4	1
14	F	64		20/63	20/25	4	3
15	M	59	PDT	20/50	20/40	20	14
16	F	57	PDT	20/40	20/30	31	17
17	F	54	PDT	20/1,600	20/1,600	31	15
18	M	45	PDT	20/60	20/40	29	10
19	M	45	PDT	20/50	20/20	26	14
20	M	41	PDT	20/20	20/20	29	6
21	F	50		20/40	20/20	31	3
22	F	58		20/400	20/400	24	1
23	M	66	PDT	20/1,000	20/200	30	5
24	F	66		20/100	20/200	24	5

Patients 1–15 were reported in the study by Finger et al. [39] and patients 16–24 were reported by Myung et al. [42].
Patients 16–19 received maintenance treatment with bimonthly injections with bevacizumab.

Patients 16–19 received a regular maintenance therapy, with injections once every 2 months. These patients had already lost their vision in the other eye, and seemed to be at a greater risk of losing vision in the treated eye. The other patients received an on-demand treatment in case of recurrent or persistent activity of the CNV, either on optical coherence tomography (OCT) examination or on FA. The number of retreatments in these patients was relatively low, starting with only 1 injection, and with a mean of 2–3 injections per year during follow-up. Four patients received only 1 injection and remained stable during 1 year. In certain patients with choroidal CNV associated with angioid streaks, intravitreal bevacizumab can restore VA and normalize the macular morphology for an extended period of time. However, most patients needed more than one treatment, and regular follow-up once every month seems to be mandatory in all patients.

Only 4 patients experienced a loss of VA, and in another 4 patients VA did not change. VA in all other patients improved. Seven patients had a VA of 20/40 or more, and none of these patients lost vision. Following treatment, 12 patients had a VA of 20/40 or more. The sooner one starts treatment at a stage of the disease with minimal abnormalities in the posterior pole, the better one is able to stop the progression of the CNV, and preserve vision. Five patients had a VA <20/200, of which 3 showed a modest improvement and the others remained the same.

Patients who received previous PDT treatment, in general, showed more extensive alterations in the posterior pole, especially larger areas of RPE atrophy, and most started with a lower VA at baseline and did not improve much (fig. 1). However, the first presentation of a CNV in patients with PXE is in most cases a classical type of CNV, with limited dimensions, and these types of CNV in general respond favorably to treatment (fig. 2). Some patients have been reported with a prolonged recurrence-free period following intravitreal treatment with bevacizumab. One patient has been reported with an improvement in VA from 20/70 to 20/20 for a period of 32 months, following three monthly injections with bevacizumab [44]. The majority of patients will experience a recurrence of the CNV, and need additional treatments. In some of these patients the recurrences are frequent and these patients need careful follow-up to prevent loss of VA. As stated, some authors think the risk of recurrence and subsequent vision loss is so great that a maintenance therapy with injections once every 2 or 3 months is justified [36, 42]. Indeed the rate of recurrence seemed to be lower in patients treated with a maintenance treatment schedule compared to those treated on demand, but both regimens were equally capable of improving or stabilizing VA and there are insufficient data at present to draw definite conclusions on the optimal dosing schedule.

Later in the course of the disease, at a time when secondary atrophic changes have occurred in the posterior pole, the CNV changes to a more occult type, with larger dimensions and a more widespread leakage. In this type of lesion the patient is generally older, the VA is already lower, and the response to treatment, even though anatomically successful, will not lead to a great improvement in VA but most of the time will stabilize vision.

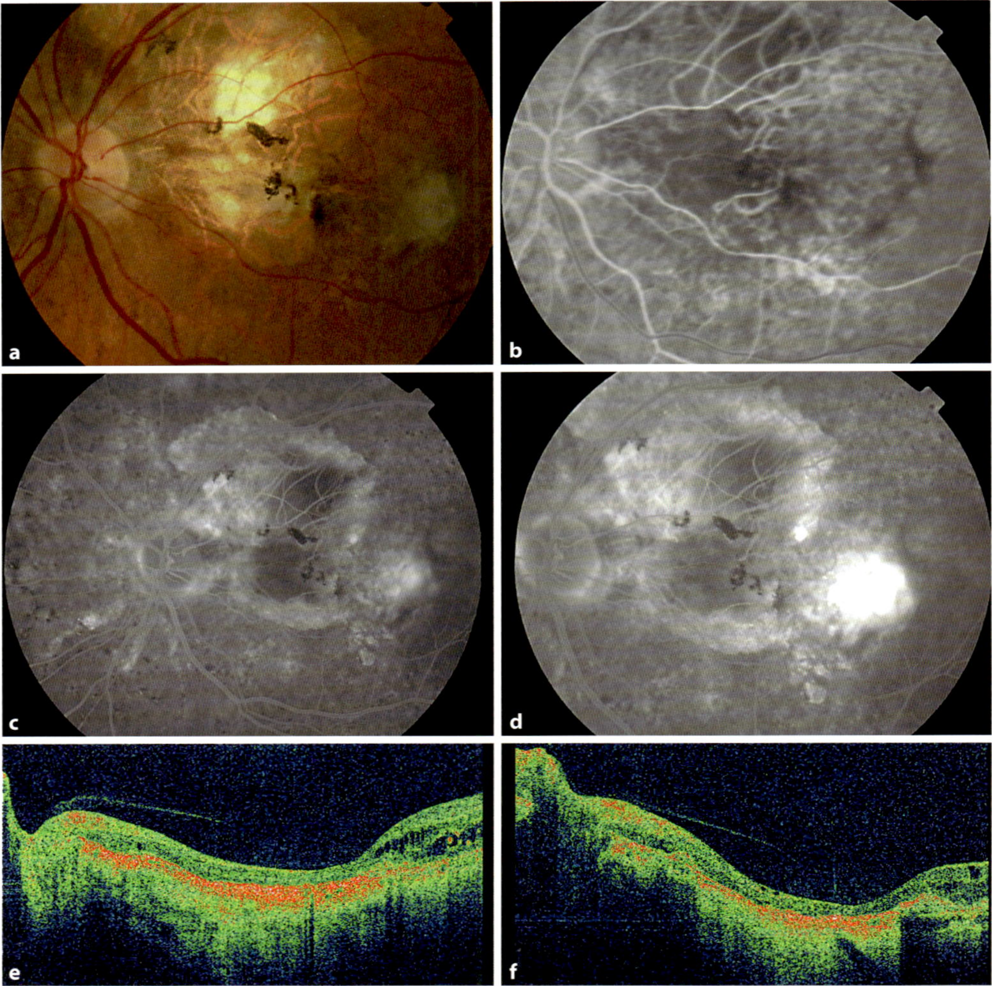

Fig. 1. Patient with late stage of ocular changes seen in PXE, previously been treated with PDT, with extended central atrophy, still active CNV temporally, without favorable response to additional three monthly injections with ranibizumab, AVOS pretreatment 20/300, and posttreatment 20/400. **a** Color fundus photograph; **b**–**d** early-, mid-, and late-phase fluorescein angiogram; **e** OCT macula before treatment with central atrophy and temporal leakage; **f** OCT same location after treatment showing no improvement.

OCT measurements reflected the favorable response seen in the patients. In the study by Myung et al. [42], the mean baseline greatest lesion height was 362 μm (median 332 μm, range 125–664 μm). At 6 months the mean greatest lesion height decreased to 201 μm (range 32–307 μm), and at the last visit further decreased to a mean of 146 μm (median 144 μm, range 73–290 μm). The reported average change of the greatest lesion height was a mean decrease of 216 μm from the first to the last

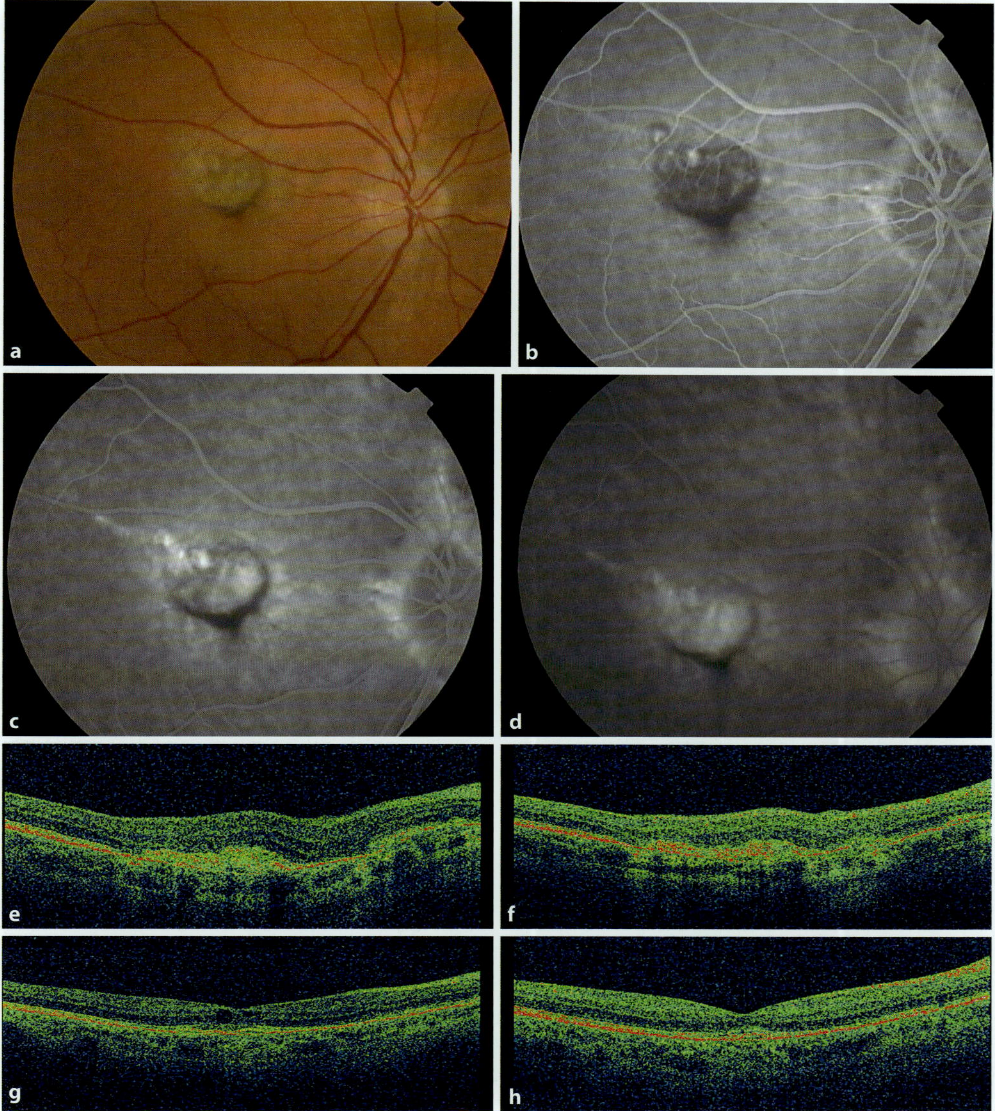

Fig. 2. Patient, 48 years of age, with early stage changes due to PXE, central macula shows no atrophy, extrafoveal neovascularization. **a** Color fundus photograph; **b–d** early-, mid- and late fluorescein angiogram; **e**, **f** OCT pretreatment showing thickened retina on top of lesion and central cystic leakage, AVOD 20/40; **g**, **h**, OCT posttreatment, 6 months following a single injection with ranibizumab, retina on top of lesion normalized and no central edema, AVOD 20/20.

OCT measurement. In the study by Finger et al. [39] all patients showed a morphological improvement following treatment, as a reduction in leakage and retinal edema demonstrated by FA and OCT, but some patients experienced further loss of vision and some did not improve as much in function as one would have expected from the morphological improvement. Treatment with bevacizumab was most efficient in patients with fewer changes at the posterior pole, at a stage where the disease process was not far progressed.

PXE patients are prone to cardiovascular events. Widespread atherosclerosis, intermittent claudicatio, angina pectoris, and early myocardial infarction belong to the spectrum of cardiovascular abnormalities seen in PXE. One of the possible side effects of intravitreal anti-VEGF therapy could be an increased risk to just these cardiovascular events, although to date no definite proof of this increased risk has been documented. In the PXE patients reported in literature, treated with anti-VEGF, no patient suffered from heart attack or stroke. One case has been described of a non-arteritic anterior optic neuropathy, occurring 2 weeks following an injection with bevacizumab in a patient with PXE, and a CNV secondary to angioid streaks [45]. However, a direct causal relationship in the presented case could neither be proven nor rejected.

Conclusions

From the present evidence it may be concluded that intravitreal anti-VEGF therapy with ranibizumab or bevacizumaab is beneficial for the treatment of CNV secondary to angioid streaks associated with PXE. The positive outcome described in the earliest studies, mostly in case series, including a limited number of patients and a relative short follow-up, were confirmed by two larger case series with follow-up of up to 2 years [39, 42].

No other treatment modality was able to reach the same positive results. Even with the most promising therapy, PDT, results were poor regarding the preservation of VA, probably to the collateral damage inherent to this treatment 30, 35]. Although there seem to be arguments to treat selected patients with a maintenance treatment of intravitreal injections once every 2 months, the majority of patients will be treated with an as-needed regimen. Unfortunately the low number of patients prevents larger controlled trials necessary to draw conclusions based on sound research. In addition, it seems to be unethical to withhold treatment in patients with CNV. A larger prospective uncontrolled clinical trial about the efficacy and safety of ranibizumab in treatment of CNV in PXE patients has been started to recruit in 2010 (PXE-CNV 06 htpp://www.clinicaltrilas.gov).

Patients need to be aware of the off-label nature of the treatment with anti-VEGF. Patients also need to be informed about the possible increased risk of cardiovascular and/or thromboembolic events, although at present no definite proof has been documented of this higher risk in patients with or without PXE treated with intravitreal anti-VEGF. Overall, based on available evidence, intravitreal treatment with anti-VEGF seems to be the best choice at present to treat patients with CNV secondary to angioid streaks and PXE.

References

1 Chassaing N, Martin L, Calvas P, Le BM, Hovnanian A: Pseudoxanthoma elasticum: a clinical, pathophysiological and genetic update including 11 novel ABCC6 mutations. J Med Genet 2005;42:881–892.

2 Finger RP, Charbel IP, Ladewig MS, Gotting C, Szliska C, Scholl HP, et al: Pseudoxanthoma elasticum: genetics, clinical manifestations and therapeutic approaches. Surv Ophthalmol 2009;54:272–285.

3 Plomp AS, Toonstra J, Bergen AA, van Dijk MR, de Jong PT: Proposal for updating the pseudoxanthoma elasticum classification system and a review of the clinical findings. Am J Med Genet A 2010; 152A:1049–1058.

4 Fabbri E, Forni GL, Guerrini G, Borgna-Pignatti C: Pseudoxanthoma-elasticum-like syndrome and thalassemia: an update. Dermatol Online J 2009;15:7.

5 Laube S, Moss C: Pseudoxanthoma elasticum. Arch Dis Child 2005;90:754–756.

6 Li Q, Jiang Q, Pfendner E, Varadi A, Uitto J: Pseudoxanthoma elasticum: clinical phenotypes, molecular genetics and putative pathomechanisms. Exp Dermatol 2009;18:1–11.

7 Bergen AA, Plomp AS, Hu X, de Jong PT, Gorgels TG: ABCC6 and pseudoxanthoma elasticum. Pflugers Arch 2007;453:685–691.

8 Pfendner EG, Vanakker OM, Terry SF, Vourthis S, McAndrew PE, McClain MR, et al: Mutation detection in the ABCC6 gene and genotype-phenotype analysis in a large international case series affected by pseudoxanthoma elasticum. J Med Genet 2007; 44:621–628.

9 Vanakker OM, Leroy BP, Coucke P, Bercovitch LG, Uitto J, Viljoen D, et al: Novel clinico-molecular insights in pseudoxanthoma elasticum provide an efficient molecular screening method and a comprehensive diagnostic flowchart. Hum Mutat 2008; 29:205.

10 Gorgels TG, Hu X, Scheffer GL, van der Wal AC, Toonstra J, de Jong PT, et al: Disruption of Abcc6 in the mouse: novel insight in the pathogenesis of pseudoxanthoma elasticum. Hum Mol Genet 2005; 14:1763–1773.

11 Zarbock R, Hendig D, Szliska C, Kleesiek K, Gotting C: Vascular endothelial growth factor gene polymorphisms as prognostic markers for ocular manifestations in pseudoxanthoma elasticum. Hum Mol Genet 2009;18:3344–3351.

12 Neldner KH: Pseudoxanthoma elasticum. Clin Dermatol 1988;6:1–159.

13 Neldner KH: Pseudoxanthoma elasticum. Int J Dermatol 1988;27:98–100.

14 Lebwohl M, Neldner K, Pope FM, De Paepe A, Christiano AM, Boyd CD, et al: Classification of pseudoxanthoma elasticum: report of a consensus conference. J Am Acad Dermatol 1994;30:103–107.

15 Lafaut BA, Priem H, De Laey JJ: Indocyanine green angiography in angioid streaks. Bull Soc Belge Ophtalmol 1997;265:21–24.

16 Lafaut BA, Leys AM, Scassellati-Sforzolini B, Priem H, De Laey JJ: Comparison of fluorescein and indocyanine green angiography in angioid streaks. Graefes Arch Clin Exp Ophthalmol 1998;236:346–353.

17 Mansour AM, Ansari NH, Shields JA, Annesley WH Jr, Cronin CM, Stock EL: Evolution of angioid streaks. Ophthalmologica 1993;207:57–61.

18 Finger RP, Charbel IP, Ladewig M, Gotting C, Holz FG, Scholl HP: Fundus autofluorescence in pseudoxanthoma elasticum. Retina 2009;29:1496–1505.

19 Hu X, Plomp AS, van SS, Wijnholds J, de Jong PT, Bergen AA: Pseudoxanthoma elasticum: a clinical, histopathological, and molecular update. Surv Ophthalmol 2003;48:424–438.

20 Mansour AM, Annesley WH: Comet-tailed drusen of the retinal pigment epithelium in angioid streaks. Eye (Lond) 1998;12:943–944.

21 Pierro L, Brancato R, Minicucci M, Pece A: Echographic diagnosis of drusen of the optic nerve head in patients with angioid streaks. Ophthalmologica 1994;208:239–242.

22 Popescu MP: Presence of choroidal neovascular membranes in pseudoxanthoma elasticum. Rev Chir Oncol Radiol ORL Oftalmol Stomatol Ser Oftalmol 1987;31:219–220.

23 Puig J, Garcia-Arumi J, Salvador F, Sararols L, Calatayud M, Alforja S: Subretinal neovascularization and hemorrhages in angioid streaks (in Spanish). Arch Soc Esp Oftalmol 2001;76:309–314.

24 Soutome N, Sugahara M, Okada AA, Hida T: Subretinal hemorrhages after blunt trauma in pseudoxanthoma elasticum. Retina 2007;27:807–808.

25 Atmaca LS, Ozmert E: Macular involvement in angioid streaks. Gronblad-Strandberg syndrome (in French). J Fr Ophtalmol 1992;15:249–253.

26 Donaldson EJ: Angioid streaks. Aust J Ophthalmol 1983;11:55–58.

27 Sato K, Ikeda T: Fluorescein angiographic features of neovascular maculopathy in angioid streaks. Jpn J Ophthalmol 1994;38:417–422.

28 Schiano LD, Parravano MC, Chiaravalloti A, Varano M: Choroidal neovascularization in angioid streaks and pseudoxanthoma elasticum: 1 year follow-up. Eur J Ophthalmol 2009;19:151–153.

29 Browning AC, Chung AK, Ghanchi F, Harding SP, Musadiq M, Talks SJ, et al: Verteporfin photodynamic therapy of choroidal neovascularization in angioid streaks: one-year results of a prospective case series. Ophthalmology 2005;112:1227–1231.
30 Chung AK, Gauba V, Ghanchi FD: Photodynamic therapy using verteporfin for juxtafoveal choroidal neovascularisation in angioid streaks associated with pseudoxanthoma elasticum: 40 months' results. Eye (Lond) 2006;20:629–631.
31 Hedaya J, Freeman WR: The effect of treatments given to patients before initiation of antivascular endothelial growth factor treatment. Retina 2008; 28:911–912.
32 Roth DB, Estafanous M, Lewis H: Macular translocation for subfoveal choroidal neovascularization in angioid streaks: Am J Ophthalmol 2001;131:390–392.
33 Singerman LJ, Hatem G: Laser treatment of choroidal neovascular membranes in angioid streaks. Retina 1981;1:75–83.
34 Tassignon MJ, Merckaert I, De CA, Cornelis MT: Treatment of choroidal neovascular membranes in a case of pseudoxanthoma elasticum (in French). Bull Soc Belge Ophtalmol 1985;214:107–112.
35 Menchini U, Virgili G, Introini U, Bandello F, Ambesi-Impiombato M, Pece A, et al: Outcome of choroidal neovascularization in angioid streaks after photodynamic therapy. Retina 2004;24:763–771.
36 Bhatnagar P, Freund KB, Spaide RF, Klancnik JM Jr, Cooney MJ, Ho I, et al: Intravitreal bevacizumab for the management of choroidal neovascularization in pseudoxanthoma elasticum. Retina 2007;27:897–902.
37 Derriman L, Marshall J, Moorman C, Downes SM: The use of intravitreal bevacizumab to treat choroidal neovascular membranes. Retina 2008;28:910–911.
38 Donati MC, Virgili G, Bini A, Giansanti F, Rapizzi E, Giacomelli G, et al: Intravitreal bevacizumab (Avastin) for choroidal neovascularization in angioid streaks: a case series. Ophthalmologica 2009;223: 24–27.
39 Finger RP, Charbel IP, Ladewig M, Holz FG, Scholl HP: Intravitreal bevacizumab for choroidal neovascularisation associated with pseudoxanthoma elasticum. Br J Ophthalmol 2008;92:483–487.
40 Japiassu RM, Japiassu MA, Pecego MG: Intravitreal bevacizumab in choroidal neovascularization secondary to Gronblad-Strandberg syndrome: case report. Arq Bras Oftalmol 2008;71:427–429.
41 Lommatzsch A: Management of choroidal vascularisation. Br J Ophthalmol 2008;92:445–446.
42 Myung JS, Bhatnagar P, Spaide RF, Klancnik JM Jr, Cooney MJ, Yannuzzi LA, et al: Long-term outcomes of intravitreal antivascular endothelial growth factor therapy for the management of choroidal neovascularisation in pseudoxanthoma elasticum. Retina 2009.
43 Rinaldi M, Dell'Omo R, Romano MR, Chiosi F, Cipollone U, Costagliola C: Intravitreal bevacizumab for choroidal neovascularization secondary to angioid streaks. Arch Ophthalmol 2007;125:1422–1423.
44 Kovach JL, Schwartz SG, Hickey M, Puliafito CA: Thirty-two month follow-up of successful treatment of choroidal neovascularization from angioid streaks with intravitreal bevacizumab. Ophthalmic Surg Lasers Imaging 2009;40:77–79.
45 Ganssauge M, Wilhelm H, Bartz-Schmidt KU, Aisenbrey S: Non-arteritic anterior ischemic optic neuropathy after intravitreal injection of bevacizumab (Avastin) for treatment of angioid streaks in pseudoxanthoma elasticum. Graefes Arch Clin Exp Ophthalmol 2009;247:1707–1710.

Frank D. Verbraak, MD, PhD
Departments of Ophthalmology and Biomedical Engineering & Physics
Academic Medical Center, Meibergdreef 9
NL–1105 AZ Amsterdam (The Netherlands)
Tel. +31 20 566 4351, E-Mail f.d.verbraak@amc.nl

Bandello F, Battaglia Parodi M (eds): Anti-VEGF.
Dev Ophthalmol. Basel, Karger, 2010, vol 46, pp 107–110

Antivascular Endothelial Growth Factor in Hereditary Dystrophies

Maurizio Battaglia Parodi[a] · Pierluigi Iacono[b] · Francesco Bandello[a]

[a]Department of Ophthalmology, University Vita-Salute, Scientific Institute San Raffaele, Milan, and [b]Fondazione G.B. Bietti per l'Oftalmologia, Istituto di Ricovero e Cura a Carattere Scientifico, Rome, Italy

Abstract

Choroidal neovascularization can rarely complicate the course of a number of chorioretinal hereditary dystrophies leading to an even further impaired vision function. In recent years, several case reports and case series have shown that intravitreal injections of antivascular endothelial growth factor drugs can be effective in treating subfoveal choroidal neovascularization secondary to chorioretinal dystrophies either improving vision, or at least halting its progressive loss. Additional studies are warranted to confirm the initial positive response and to assess the best therapeutic regimen.

Choroidal neovascularization (CNV) can rarely complicate the course of several chorioretinal dystrophies. Little is known regarding the natural history of this form of CNV. Visual acuity (VA) can be stable for a long time with a late evolution toward fibrosis and atrophy [1]. Nevertheless, the occurrence of a CNV, especially with subfoveal location, is often associated with a visual function deterioration. Some authors have employed laser photocoagulation and photodynamic therapy to reverse or halt the consequent visual impairment, achieving limited beneficial effects [2, 3]. The advent of therapy based on intravitreal injection of antivascular endothelial growth factor drugs has brought new hope in the treatment of this complication of chorioretinal dystrophies. Additional studies are warranted to confirm the initial positive response and to assess the best therapeutic regimen.

Best's Dystrophy

Two reports have described a positive effect of intravitreal injections of both bevacizumab and ranibizumab for the treatment of a subfoveal CNV related to vitelliform

Best's disease [4, 5]. In both cases, optical coherence tomography (OCT) examination revealed the complete resolution of the sensory retinal detachment, over a short-term follow-up. Bearing in mind the young age of patients affected by Best vitelliform dystrophy, this approach could be extremely beneficial for visual prognosis and quality of life.

Pattern Dystrophy

A single report describes a case of adult-onset foveomacular vitelliform dystrophy associated and complicated by occult CNV who underwent intravitreal bevacizumab with progressive decrease of subretinal fluid, but with no VA improvement [6].

Our experience includes 8 patients affected by subfoveal CNV associated with pattern dystrophy of the retinal pigment epithelium, who were treated with intravitreal bevacizumab and prospectively followed up for 24 months. The mean best corrected VA (BCVA) and the mean foveal thickness (FT) at baseline were 0.73 ± 0.37 (logMAR ± SD) and 281 ± 104 μm (CMT ± SD), respectively. At the 3-month examination, mean BCVA improved significantly to 0.52 ± 0.29 and mean FT decreased to 222 ± 78 μm. Subsequently, at the 6- and 12-month examinations, a substantial stabilization of the mean BCVA was observed, whereas the mean FT changed to 217 ± 52 and 208 ± 58 μm, respectively. At the final visit, mean BCVA showed a statistically significant improvement of 2.4 lines in comparison to the baseline value. The mean FT finally decreased to 197 ± 36 μm.

Overall, a mean number of 4.4 intravitreal bevacizumab injections was administered during the 24 months of follow-up. No side effect or complication was registered during the follow-up period. On the basis of our practice, we believe that intravitreal injection of bevacizumab can be regarded as a beneficial treatment for pattern dystrophy-related subfoveal CNV. Further studies are necessary to assess the best therapeutic regimen and the most appropriate monitoring procedures.

Intravitreal injection of bevacizumab was performed in a case affected by adult-onset vitelliform dystrophy with no evidence of CNV [7]. During 4 months of follow-up the spectral domain OCT showed a progressive decrease of yellowish deposits and complete resolution of subretinal fluid which accompanied the lipofuscin-like material. Unfortunately, a mild decrease in VA and persistence of metamorphopsia was registered.

Retinitis Pigmentosa

Some authors have recently reported on the use of intravitreal bevacizumab to treat cystoid macular edema complicating retinitis pigmentosa. This complication occurs in about 20% of cases [8] and oral carbonic anhydrase inhibitors have been reported as the most effective treatment to manage it.

A former interventional case series of 2 eyes treated with intravitreal bevacizumab injections demonstrated the absence of a positive effect [9], whereas another interventional case series including 13 eyes of 7 patients revealed a progressive reduction of the central macular thickness in association with visual function improvement [10]. Positive results have also been reported in a single case of CME secondary to a poor response to oral acetazolamide and following treatment with pegaptanib intravitreal injection [11].

Further studies with a larger population and longer follow-up period are warranted to assess the efficacy of this approach.

Fundus Flavimaculatus

A single case of fundus flavimaculatus associated with CNV was submitted to intravitreal ranibizumab injections at monthly intervals. Six months after three injections, VA improved from 20/64 to 20/32, with resolution of serous retinal detachment on OCT [12]. This case report indicates that intravitreal ranibizumab may be considered a possible valuable therapeutic option for this rare association.

Sorsby Fundus Dystrophy

A case of CNV secondary to genetically demonstrated Sorsby fundus dystrophy was treated with three initial intravitreal injections of bevacizumab at a dose of 5 mg/kg at 2-week intervals, followed by an additional injection because of CNV recurrence at the 7-month follow-up [13]. After 16 months of follow-up, VA had improved from 20/50 at baseline to 20/25, whereas OCT and fluorescein angiography showed no evidence of CNV activity.

References

1 Parodi MB: Eredodistrofie Corioretiniche. Rome, Verduci Editore, 2002.
2 Parodi MB: Choroidal neovascularization in fundus pulverulentus. Acta Ophthalmol Scand 2002;80:559–560.
3 Parodi MB, Liberali T, Pedio M, Francis PJ, Piccolino FC, Fiotti N, Romano M, Ravalico G: Photodynamic therapy of subfoveal choroidal neovascularization secondary to reticular pattern dystrophy: three-year results of an uncontrolled, prospective case series. Am J Ophthalmol 2006;141:1152–1154.
4 Querques G, Bocco MCA, Soubrane G, Souied EH: Intravitreal ranibizumab (Lucentis) for choroidal neovascularisation associated with vitelliform macular dystrophy. Acta Ophthalmol 2008;86:694–695.
5 Leu J, Schrage NF, Degenring RF: Choroidal neovascularisation secondary to Best's disease in a 13-year-old boy treated by intravitreal Bevacizumab. Graefes Arch Clin Exp Ophthalmol 2007;245:1723–1725.
6 Montero JA, Ruiz-Moreno JM, De La Vega C: Intravitreal bevacizumab for adult-onset vitelliform dystrophy: a case report. Eur J Ophthalmol 2007;17: 983–986.

7 Lee JY, Lim J, Chung H, Kim JG, Yoon YH: Spectral domain optical coherence tomography in a patient with adult-onset vitelliform dystrophy treated with intravitreal bevacizumab. Ophthalmic Surg Lasers Imaging 2009;40:319–321.
8 Fishman JA, Maggiano JM, Fishman M: Foveal lesions seen in retinitis pigmentosa. Arch Ophthalmol 1977;95:1993–1996.
9 Melo GB, Farah ME, Aggio FB: Intravitreal injection of bevacizumab for cystoid macular edema in retinitis pigmentosa. Acta Ophthalmol 2007;85:461–463.
10 Yuzbasioglu E, Artunay O, Rasier R, Sengul A, Bahcecioglu H: Intravitreal bevacizumab (Avastin) injection in retinitis pigmentosa. Curr Eye Res 2009; 34:231–237.
11 Querques G, Prascina F, Iaculli C, et al: Intravitreal pegaptanib sodium (Macugen) for refractory cystoid macular edema in pericentral retinitis pigmentosa. Int Ophthalmol 2009;29:103–107.
12 Quijano C, Querques G, Massamba N, Soubrane G, Souied EH: Type 3 choroidal neovascularization associated with fundus flavimaculatus. Ophthalmic Res 2009;42:152–154.
13 Prager F, Michels S, Geitzenauer W, Schmidt-Erfurth U: Choroidal neovascularization secondary to Sorsby fundus dystrophy treated with systemic bevacizumab (Avastin). Acta Ophthalmol Scand 2007;85:904–906.

Francesco Bandello, MD, FEBO
Professor and Chairman, Department of Ophthalmology
University Vita-Salute Scientific Institute, San Raffaele
Via Olgettina, 60, IT–20132 Milan (Italy)
Tel. +39 02 2643 2648, Fax +39 02 2648 3643, E-Mail francesco.bandello@hsr.it

Bandello F, Battaglia Parodi M (eds): Anti-VEGF.
Dev Ophthalmol. Basel, Karger, 2010, vol 46, pp 111–122

Antivascular Endothelial Growth Factor as an Approach for Macular Edema

P.M. Buchholz · A.P. Buchholz · A.J. Augustin

Augenklinik, Karlsruhe, Germany

Abstract

Macular edema is an abnormal thickening of the macula associated with the accumulation of excess fluid in the extracellular space of the neurosensory retina. The following chapter looks at the basic pathomechanisms of macular edema as well as major pathologic conditions leading to it: special focus is on diabetic retinopathy, retinal venous occlusions and a number of inflammatory disorders. Currently available data on up-to-date pharmacologic treatment options such as steroids and anti-VEGF compounds is presented and discussed.

Broadly defined, macular edema (ME) is an abnormal thickening of the macula associated with the accumulation of excess fluid in the extracellular space of the neurosensory retina. Intracellular edema involving Müller cells has also been observed histopathologically in some cases. The term cystoid macular edema (CME) applies when there is evidence by biomicroscopy, fluorescein angiography (FA) and/or optical coherence tomography (OCT) of fluid accumulation into multiple cyst-like spaces within the macula.

Several basic pathophysiologic processes may contribute to the development of ME, which occurs in association with a wide variety of pathologic conditions. ME presents the final common pathway in many prevalent retinal disorders and can be considered the leading cause of central vision loss in the developed world. It is thus of markedly medical and socioeconomic importance.

Since the pathogenesis of ME depends on the underlying etiology and because it may be multifactorial, an effective management is based upon recognizing and addressing each factor that is expressed in a given clinical setting. The treatment of ME has evolved dramatically over the past two decades. Research has led to a better understanding of its causes, but also to the development of new therapeutic options [1].

Basic Pathophysiologic Mechanisms

Normally, volume and composition of the extracellular compartment of the neurosensory retina and subretinal space is regulated by retinal capillary endothelial cell and retinal pigment epithelium (RPE) tight junctions as well as the pumping functions of RPE cells. However, if there is a loss of function in such fluid barriers or effective RPE pump mechanisms, intraretinal fluid will accumulate. OCT imaging reveals that ME is located mostly in the outer retinal layers [2]. Most commonly, ME is a result of pathologic hyperpermeability of retinal blood vessels. Increased vascular permeability leads to extravasation of fluid, proteins and other molecules into the retinal interstitium. Depending on the underlying disease, the latter may include prostaglandins, leukotrienes, protein kinase C, nitric oxide and various cytokines such as vascular endothelial growth factor (VEGF), TNF-α and interleukins.

Clinically leakage from retinal blood vessels is best detected with FA, while OCT imaging is a sensitive method for detecting and quantifying macular thickening regardless of its cause. Leakage of fluid is further enhanced by factors that increase retinal blood flow such as vasodilation, rising intraluminal pressure and increasing blood volume. Additionally there is evidence that alterations in the outer blood-retinal (RPE) barrier may contribute directly to ME in conditions such as diabetic retinopathy and postoperative states [1]. Furthermore, tractional stress by perifoveal vitreous detachment or epiretinal membrane as well as various abnormalities causing fluid leakage from the optic nerve head can lead to intraretinal fluid accumulation and ME. Regardless of the pathogenic mechanisms causing ME, the resulting loss in visual acuity (VA) essentially depends on macular thickening and various other factors such as duration of edema, perfusion of macular capillaries, photoreceptor impairment, dysfunction and media opacities [2].

Major Pathologic Conditions Leading to ME: Retinal Vascular Disease

Diabetic Retinopathy

DME is the leading cause of vision loss in patients with diabetes. It occurs in diabetes types 1 and 2 and increases in incidence with the severity of diabetic retinopathy. Chronic hyperglycemia is a major initiator of microvascular complications in diabetes. It sets off a series of metabolic events, stimulating the expressions of multiple cytokines such as VEGF and produces vascular dysfunction and damage that includes loss of endothelial cells, increased permeability and leukocyte adhesion and alterations in blood flow leading to diabetic retinopathy and potentially diabetic macular edema (DME).

The prevalence of diabetic retinopathy is available from major European countries and the USA. According to a survey published in Germany in 2000, the prevalence of diabetic retinopathy was estimated at 22% in diabetic patients [3]. Data from a study carried out in 2002 by the University of Valladolid in Spain gave a similar prevalence (20.9%) with regard to retinopathy in diabetic patients [4]. In the UK, up to 10% of people with diabetes will have retinopathy requiring ophthalmologic follow-up or treatment [5]. It has been estimated that if untreated, 6–9% of patients with proliferative retinopathy or severe non-proliferative retinopathy will become blind each year [6]. Within the Wisconsin Epidemiologic Study of Diabetic Retinopathy (WESDR), a population-based study from a well-defined area, researchers found a prevalence of 71% for diabetic retinopathy in a group of 996 patients who were below the age of 30 at onset of diabetes [7]. Data on incidence is much more limited. In Germany for example, 2.13% of diabetics are estimated to develop diabetic retinopathy each year [5]. The WESDR reported an incidence of 59% over a 4-year interval [8].

The prevalence of DME has also been recorded. In Spain, out of 20.9% of diabetic patients with retinopathy, ME was found in 5.7% [4]. In the UK, there are an estimated 380,000 blind people and 579,000 partially sighted people. According to the Royal College of Ophthalmologists of London, ME is responsible for 70% of visual loss in diabetic patients [5]. The prevalence of ME in the WESDR, severe enough to be a likely cause of visual disturbance, ranged between 4 and 11%. Based on these data it was estimated (as of 1993) that of approximately 7,800,000 people in North America with diabetes, 84,000 would develop proliferative retinopathy and about 95,000 would develop ME over a 10-year period [9].

The pathophysiology of ME in diabetic eyes is complex. Increases in retinal blood flow may partly explain the extravasation of fluid into the extracellular compartment, the most important mechanism however is the breakdown of the blood-retinal barriers. VEGF is a highly potent vasopermeability factor and has demonstrated to play a major role in this process. In the past, focal laser photocoagulation has been the only proven treatment as well as standard of care in patients with clinically significant DME. Pharmacologic therapies are usually considered in eyes with perfused, non-tractional, diffuse DME which is refractory and unlikely to respond to laser treatment [1].

Retinal Venous Occlusions

An immediate consequence of retinal venous thrombosis is elevation of the intravascular pressure in retinal veins distal to the occlusion site. The breakdown of the blood-retinal barrier in hypoxic retina is mediated by upregulated cytokines such as VEGF, which causes leakage of fluids and proteins. By these mechanisms both central retinal vein occlusions (CRVO) and branch retinal vein occlusions (BRVO) commonly result in ME which tends to be chronic, difficult to treat and visually disabling [1]. A recent study has also highlighted that a reduction in perifoveal capillary blood-flow velocity may be involved in the development of ME in patients with BRVO [10].

A recent survey found that few epidemiology data are available for BRVO as well as CRVO. BRVO is the second most common retinal vascular disorder after diabetic retinopathy [11]. There were no European population-based studies identified in literature. Such studies however are needed to better understand the epidemiology of RVO in Europe and yield reliable, valid, generalizable incidence and prevalence estimates of BRVO and CRVO. It was concluded that from available material the Beaver Dam Eye Study currently provides the best estimate [12]. The Beaver Dam Eye Study found a prevalence and incidence for BRVO of 0.6 an 0.12% respectively. Furthermore, the study showed a respective prevalence and incidence for CRVO of 0.1 and 0.04% [13].

Based on the findings from the Beaver Dam Eye Study, the following extrapolations suggest that prevalence of BRVO ranges from 130,000 (Spain) to 270,000 cases (Germany), and incidence from 26,000 to 54,000 cases. For CRVO, prevalence ranges from 22,000 and 45,000 cases and incidence from 9,000 to 18,000 cases [12]. Following a CRVO or BRVO incident, vision loss is often exacerbated by macular hemorrhage, macular ischemia or submacular fluid with secondary RPE damage. In randomized clinical trials, grid laser treatment has shown to produce at least modest visual benefit in eyes with BRVO, however not in cases of CRVO. There are thus very limited treatment options in CRVO. In recent times, pharmacologic therapies have been introduced as alternative approaches for treatment of vein occlusions [1].

Inflammatory Disorders

Several different underlying inflammatory disorders also result in ME as a common phenotype.

CME following cataract surgery (Irvine-Gass syndrome) can be detected by FA and remains the most common cause of visual loss in this setting. While it occurs in approximately 20% of uncomplicated cases, it will only cause significant decrease in VA in 1–2% of operated eyes. Risk of developing postoperative CME is substantially greater in patients with preexisting conditions known to produce vasoactive stimuli such as diabetic retinopathy and uveitis [1].

A recent pilot study has demonstrated the positive correlation of VEGF concentration in aqueous samples with clinically meaningful changes in central subfield thickness measured by OCT in a subpopulation of diabetic patients undergoing cataract surgery. To further elucidate the relationship, more research is warranted [14].

The development of ME is also a known complication of laser procedures such as panretinal photocoagulation for retinal vascular disease (e.g. diabetic retinopathy, vein occlusion). Although the mechanism is not clearly understood, laser-induced inflammatory mediators such as VEGF and transudation from increased macular blood flow may play a significant role. In addition, the usage of other types of laser procedures, such as YAG laser procedures, may also enhance occurrence of CME.

CME is the most frequent complication in uveitis. It typically develops in patients with intermediate and posterior uveitis components. It may occur in a wide variety of uveitis syndromes, whether they are caused by underlying autoimmune diseases (pars planitis) or infectious (toxoplasmosis), toxic (rifabutin-associated) or idiopathic (sarcoidosis) etiologies. In all these conditions the most important pathogenic mechanism is loss of inner blood-retinal barrier integrity caused by inflammatory mediators like VEGF, which are generated by the underlying uveitic process [1].

Pharmacologic Treatment Options in ME with a Focus on Anti-VEGF Therapies

Diabetic Macular Edema
Options to treat DME effectively have not been too numerous. Apart from different types of laser treatments – which present the standard of care in treatment of DME – surgical management in the form of vitrectomy has also played a role in cases unresponsive to laser treatment.

In the category of pharmacological treatment approaches, mainly corticosteroids have been applied in the past. Corticosteroids are well-known potent anti-inflammatory compounds. Additionally they possess strong antiangiogenesis effects, also acting by suppressing VEGF gene activity and its metabolic pathway. Especially intravitreally applied triamcinolone (IVTA) has been employed with a fair number of randomized controlled clinical trials demonstrating significant improvement in DME and VA [15]. However many of the trials had small numbers of participants as well as short follow-up time periods. Also, since no IVTA compound has obtained marketing approval for the treatment of ME, concentrations and dosing schedules of triamcinolone varied across trials (e.g. 4 up to 25 mg), making comparisons in terms of efficacy and safety a challenge. The most common choice however seems to be the 4-mg concentration. Substantial adverse events were recorded in most trials, among them infections, glaucoma and cataract formation [16]. A study performed by the Diabetic Retinopathy Clinical Research (DRCR) Network investigators compared the efficacy and safety of focal/grid laser photocoagulation compared to IVTA doses of 1 or 4 mg respectively over a time period of 2 years. While at 4 months the VA in steroid-treated subjects was better than in the laser group, the difference was no more apparent in the long term. From 16 months to 2 years, laser-treated patients had better vision. These findings show that longer-term data need to be generated for the treatment of DME to determine the most effective treatment in specific patient populations [17].

More recently, intravitreal implants have been developed. These allow a more precise titration as well as extended duration of drug delivery. Examples of licensed compounds are a surgically implanted fluocinolone acetonide device as well as an injectable, biodegradable dexamethasone-loaded matrix. Data available report on improvements of VA and macular thickness, but also on steroid-typical adverse effects as previously seen with IVTA [18].

Although many agents in development inhibit the production of VEGF, research has also focused on agents that can antagonize circulating ocular VEGF. The majority of VEGF antagonists are in active development for retinal neovascularization disorders such as age-related macular degeneration. However, by virtue of the

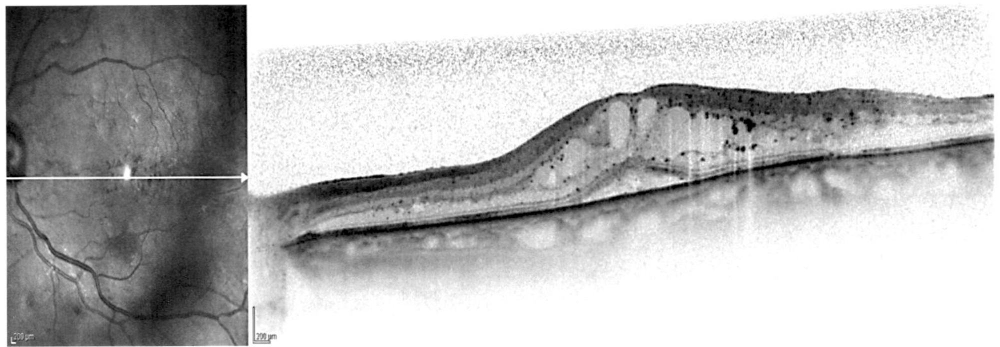

Fig. 1. Spectralis OCT of a DME patient before anti-VEGF treatment (courtesy of Anat Loewenstein, Department of Ophthalmology, Tel Aviv Medical Centre, Israel).

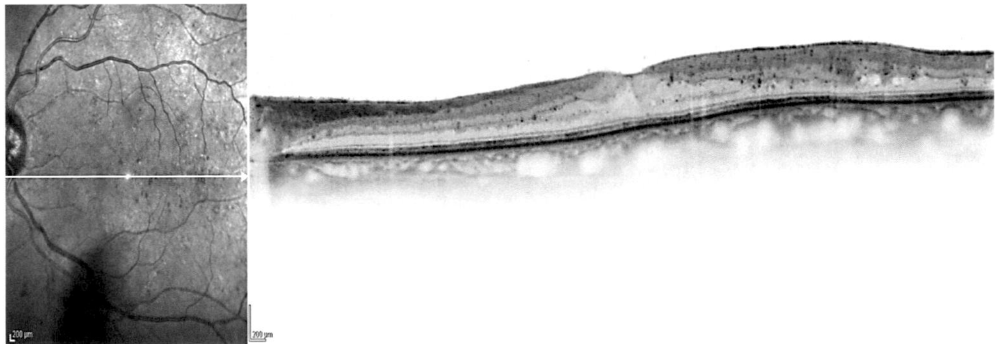

Fig. 2. Spectralis OCT of the same DME patient after anti-VEGF treatment (courtesy of Anat Loewenstein, Department of Ophthalmology, Tel Aviv Medical Centre, Israel).

common VEGF-mediated pathways that result in diabetic retinopathy and/or DME, these indications are logical additional targets for those same anti-VEGF agents (fig. 1, 2).

Unlike antiangiogenesis agents, which inhibit the production of VEGF through enzymatic or other processes, VEGF antagonists are a heterogeneous group of drugs in development that bind to free VEGF and render it unable to activate receptors in the retinal vasculature (or theoretically in any body tissue). Agents that can be classified into this group include receptor fusion proteins, anti-VEGF aptamers, and monoclonal antibodies. Though different in composition and structure, all VEGF antagonists share the ability to mimic endogenous VEGF receptors and thus 'capture' the molecule and render it inactive.

In recent years, antiangiogenic agents such as pegaptanib, bevacizumab and ranibizumab have been injected intravitreally for the treatment of choroidal neovascularization (CNV). Pegaptanib and ranibizumab have been licensed for this indication, while bevacizumab is officially licensed for use in colorectal cancer and being used off-label in ocular delivery [19].

Ranibizumab is a humanized monoclonal antibody fragment that binds to all VEGF-A isoforms of VEGF, thereby preventing binding of VEGF-A to receptors VEGFR-1 and -2 [20]. It is injected intravitreally. VEGF-A inhibition has been shown to decrease ME and retinal edema associated with CNV. A phase 2 randomized controlled clinical study evaluating efficacy and safety over 12 months in 152 DME patients receiving either 0.3 or 0.5 mg ranibizumab or sham every 4 weeks over 6 months (RESOLVE) demonstrated a significantly better efficacy of ranibizumab in terms of reducing CRT and increasing VA, while there seemed to be no notable difference between both active concentrations. A three-arm phase 3 study (RESTORE) in approximately 320 patients over 12 months is currently ongoing determining efficacy and safety of 0.5 mg ranibizumab monotherapy compared to combinations of 0.5 mg ranibizumab/sham laser and sham injection/grid laser respectively. Results are expected in 2010. Additional long-term studies (36 months) in DME (RISE, RIDE) will most likely be available in 2012 [21].

A recent study compared ranibizumab with focal/grid laser or a combination of both in 126 patients with DME. During a span of 6 months, ranibizumab injections alone had a significantly better visual outcome than laser treatment alone or a combination of both. This also applied to reduction of excess foveal thickness [22].

Bevacizumab seems to show similar efficacy to ranibizumab in treatment of CNV in AMD. It has attracted interest because of its low cost. However, systemic safety is a concern. The US National Eye Institute carried out an 18-week phase 2 trial in 121 patients with DME, which were randomized to five groups and treated with focal photocoagulation, intravitreous bevacizumab 1.25 mg, intravitreous bevacizumab 2.25 mg, intravitreous bevacizumab/combination with focal photocoagulation as well as intravitreous bevacizumab/sham respectively. Bevacizumab groups had a better reduction in central macular thickness and better median VA compared to the photocoagulation group. Differences between both bevacizumab concentrations were not meaningful. Combining bevacizumab with focal photocoagulation resulted in no apparent short-term benefit or adverse outcomes [23].

Pegaptanib is also injected intravitreally for the treatment of AMD and of DME. Pegaptanib is an anti-VEGF aptamer, a synthetic oligonucleotide with high affinity and selectivity for the isoform 165 of VEGF. A randomized controlled clinical trial in 172 DME patients who received either repeated doses of intravitreal pegaptanib or sham injections showed that treated eyes were more likely to have an improvement in VA of 10 letters or more (34 vs. 10%) as well as a reduction of macular thickness and less need for focal laser therapy at 36 weeks [24].

Essentially, studies so far did not distinguish between diffuse ME and CME. The potential benefits of doing so remain to be established [17]. Up to this point in time, clinical experience and existing studies suggest that the response of DME to intravitreal injection of anti-VEGF drugs is transient, variable and of modest magnitude in most patients. Proof of long-term efficacy and safety will require large phase III clinical trials. Such studies should also address whether this relative short-term efficacy could be extended over a longer time by combination with subsequent laser photocoagulation [1].

ME Secondary to CRVO and BRVO

Similar to the situation in diabetic retinopathy and ME, available therapeutic options have been scarce, especially in the management of CRVO. Hemodilution measures as part of a hospitalization approach have displayed large variations and employed multiple agents, making a generalized recommendation difficult [25]. The only randomized study investigating the effect of hemodilution in an outpatient setting in CRVO showed no significant benefit [26].

Effectiveness of laser treatment in ME was investigated as part of the Central Retinal Vein Occlusion Study. Data demonstrated that grid photocoagulation was not effective in improving VA in eyes with ME secondary to perfused CRVO, although there was a trend in patients younger than 60 years [27]. While the short-term results of intravitreal triamcinolone treatment of ME secondary to CRVO appear to be promising, anatomical and visual improvements seem to be often transient; safety and efficacy have so far only been shown for a specific concentration in one controlled clinical study. The SCORE (Standard Care versus Corticosteroid for Retinal Vein Occlusion) Study is a multicenter phase 3 study in 630 patients with ME in CRVO randomized to intravitreal triamcinolone 4- or 1-mg injections respectively or standard care (observation). Intravitreal triamcinolone was shown to be superior to observation for treating vision loss associated with ME. The 1-mg dose had a safety profile superior to that of the 4-mg dose. The authors suggest that intravitreal triamcinolone in a 1-mg dose, following the retreatment criteria applied in the SCORE Study, should be considered for up to 1 year, and possibly 2 years, for patients with characteristics similar to those in the SCORE-CRVO trial [28]. A trial in which patients received a dexamethasone implant containing either 350 or 700 μg has also been finalized. The results have not yet been published [29].

Several case series show that intravitreal anti-VEGF therapy may cause decrease in macular thickness and improvement in VA [19], however the reported follow-up series are short and no recommendations can be made at present [18]. Results of a currently ongoing phase 3 trial (CRUISE) are awaited in 2010. The study compares the efficacy and safety of monthly administered 0.5 or 0.3 mg ranibizumab or sham injections for a period of 6 months followed by another 6 months of observation in 390 patients. Another ongoing study (ROCC) is investigating the efficacy and safety of ranibizumab 10-mg intravitreal injections every 3 months compared to sham [19].

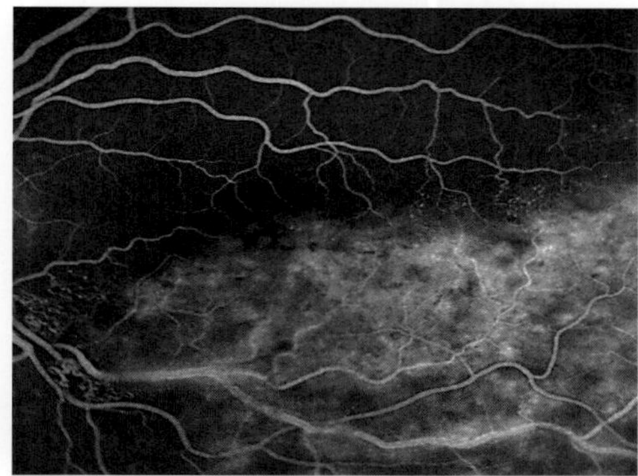

Fig. 3. Fluorescein angiogram (6 min 1 s) of a 54-year-old female patient with hypertension and an incident of BRVO.

In the case of ME secondary to BRVO there are slightly more therapeutic options at hand. The gold standard for treatment is not observation, but rather laser treatment. A randomized clinical study, the Branch Vein Occlusion Study, has demonstrated that the use of grid pattern laser photocoagulation in the distribution of leaking capillaries is beneficial if applied after a period of 3–6 months following the initial event and following absorption of the majority of hemorrhage in patients whose VA is 0.5 or worse [30].

Again, results of intravitreal triamcinolone treatment for ME secondary to BRVO appear to be promising, but so far most have not been demonstrated for a specific concentration in a controlled clinical study. Once more only the results of the SCORE (Standard Care versus Corticosteroid for Retinal Vein Occlusion) are available to give more insight. There was no difference identified in VA at 12 months for the standard care group (laser photocoagulation) compared with the triamcinolone groups, however rates of adverse events (particularly elevated intraocular pressure and cataract) were highest in the 4-mg group. The authors concluded that grid photocoagulation as applied in the SCORE Study remains the standard care for patients with vision loss associated with ME secondary to BRVO and should remain the benchmark against which other treatments are compared in clinical trials for eyes with vision loss associated with ME secondary to BRVO [31]. Results from a clinical study, where a dexamethasone implant (350 or 700 μg) was injected intravitreally in patients with ME secondary to BRVO, are not yet publicly available [32].

Currently, increasing short-term data support the fact that multiple intravitreal bevacizumab injections reduce ME secondary to BRVO, including those that had previously failed laser treatment (fig. 3, 4). The most common treatment regimen is 2–3 injections over the first 5–6 months [33]. Nevertheless, further randomized controlled trials are required to assess long-term safety [19]. A randomized controlled clinical study (BRAVO) looking at the efficacy and safety of ranibizumab 0.5 or 0.3 mg respectively, versus sham in ME secondary to BRVO, is currently being carried

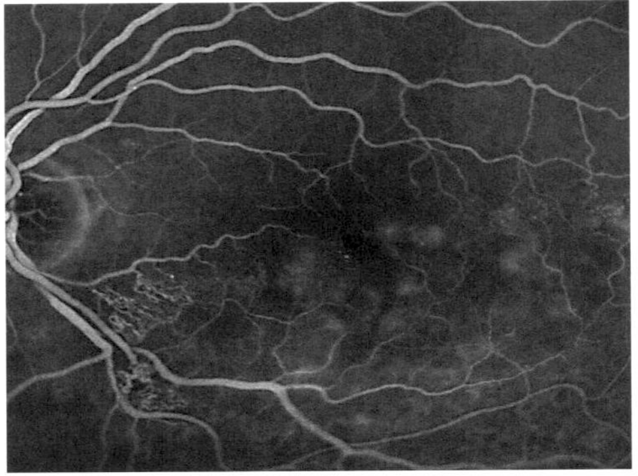

Fig. 4. Fluorescein angiogram (7 min 38 s) of the same 54-year-old female patient after anti-VEGF therapy (week 6).

out. 390 patients will be treated monthly for a 6-month period and then observed for another 6 months. Results are due in 2010 [34].

Inflammatory CME

Anti-inflammatory therapy, administered in a stepwise approach, is the mainstay of treating postoperative and uveitic CME. Pseudophakic and aphakic CME usually responds well to topical therapy with corticosteroid and non-steroidal anti-inflammatory agents. Resistant cases of postoperative CME as well as most cases of uveitic CME require higher macular concentrations, usually achieved through sub-Tenon or intravitreal injections [1]. An implant containing 0.59 mg fluocinolone acetonide demonstrated efficacy in patients with chronic non-infectious posterior uveitis and is now licensed in this indication [35]. A dexamethasone posterior-segment drug delivery system has been tested in a randomized, prospective, single-masked, controlled trial to determine efficacy and safety in treating ME resulting from uveitis or Irvine-Gass syndrome over 3 months. The results showed that in patients with persistent ME, the 700-μg concentration of dexamethasone drug delivery system was well tolerated and produced statistically significant improvements in VA and fluorescein leakage [36]. Preliminary data also suggest that intravitreal anti-VEGF therapy with bevacizumab may be associated with anatomic and visual improvement in uveitis patients with CME. Results demonstrated that despite its limited inflammatory activity, VEGF may play a role in this pathogenesis. After patients had received a single 2.5-mg intravitreal injection of bevacizumab, short-term improvement of VA and decrease of OCT retinal thickness were recorded [37]. Another study looked at the efficacy of 1.25 or 2.5 mg intravitreally applied bevacizumab for the treatment of refractory CME after cataract surgery. Again, results suggest that it is well tolerated and that treated eyes showed a significant improvement in VA as well as decrease in macular thickness by OCT at 12 months [38].

Nevertheless, to substantiate these encouraging initial results, additional controlled randomized trials will be necessary. The interest is now focusing on trials that evaluate combination therapies and/or direct comparisons between treatments. Finally, clinical experience and the actual oxygen supply will lead the physician to an individualized treatment in this complicated disease entity.

References

1 Johnson M: Perspective – etiology and treatment of macular edema. Am J Ophthalmol 2009;147:11–16.

2 Catier A, Tadayoni R: Characterization of macular edema from various etiologies by optical coherence tomography. Am J Ophthalmol 2005;140:200–206.

3 Zietz B, Kasparbauer A, Ottman S, Spiegel D, Palitzsch KD: Diabetic retinopathy and associated risk factors in type 1 and type 2 diabetics in the upper palatinate (in German). Dtsch Med Wochenschr 2000;125:783–788.

4 López IM, Diez A, Velilla S, Rueda A, Alvarez A, Pastor CJ: Prevalence of diabetic retinopathy and eye care in a rural area of Spain. Institute of Applied Ophthalmobiology (IOBA), University of Valladolid, Valladolid, Spain. Ophthalmic Epidemiol 2002;205–214.

5 Hayward LM, Burden ML, Burden AC, Blackledge H, Raymond NT, Botha JL, Karwakowski WSS, Duke T, Chang YF: What is the prevalence of visual impairment in the general and diabetic population: Are there ethnic and gender differences? Diabet Med 2002;19:27–34.

6 Philipps RP, Clearkin L: Screening for diabetic retinopathy: an overview; in Somdutt Prasad, MS, FRCS, Fellow in Diabetic Eye Disease: Arrowe Park Hospital. Upton, Wirral. The Problem of Diabetic Retinopathy: NHS NSC Diabetic Retinopathy Screening (http://www.diabetic-retinopathy.screening.nhs.uk/diabetic-retinopathy.html).

7 Klein R, Klein B: The Wisconsin Epidemiologic Study of Diabetic Retinopathy. II. Prevalence and risk of diabetic retinopathy when age at diagnosis is less than 30 years. Arch Ophthalmol 1984;102:520–526.

8 Klein R, Klein B: The Wisconsin Epidemiologic Study of Diabetic Retinopathy. XIV. Ten-year incidence and progression of diabetic retinopathy. Arch Ophthalmol 1994;112:1217–1228.

9 Klein B, Klein R: Diabetic retinopathy; in Johnson GJ, Minassian DC (eds): The Epidemiology of Eye Disease. New York, Oxford University Press, 2003, pp 342–345.

10 Noma H, Funatsu H: Macular microcirculation and macular edema in branch retinal vein occlusion. Br J Ophthalmol 2009;93:630–633.

11 Rehak J, Rehak M: Branch retinal vein occlusions: pathogenesis, visual prognosis, and treatment modalities. Curr Eye Res 2008;33:111–131.

12 Soubrane G, Buchholz P, Mahabhashyam S: The epidemiology of retinal vein occlusions in Europe: a literature review of existing data. Euretina Annual Meeting, Nice, France 2009.

13 Klein R: The epidemiology of retinal vein occlusion: the Beaver Dam Eye Study. Trans Am Ophthalmol Soc 2000;98:133–141.

14 Hartnett E, Tinkham N: Aqueous vascular endothelial growth factor as a predictor of macular thickening following cataract surgery in patients with diabetes mellitus. Am J Ophthalmol 2009;148:895–901.

15 Jonas JB, Kreissig I, Söfker A, Degenering RF: Intravitreal injection of triamcinolone for diffuse diabetic macular edema. Arch Ophthalmol 2003; 121:57–61.

16 O'Doherty M, Dooley I: Interventions for diabetic macular edema: a systematic review of the literature. Br J Ophthalmol 2008;92:1585–1587.

17 Diabetic Retinopathy Clinical Research Network: A randomized trial comparing intravitreal triamcinolone acetonide and focal/grid photocoagulation for diabetic macular edema. Ophthalmology 2008;115: 1447–1459.

18 Royal College of Ophthalmologists: Retinal vein occlusion (RVO) interim guidelines. February 2009, pp 15–16.

19 NHS UK – National Horizon Scanning Centre: Ranibizumab for macular oedema secondary to central or branch retinal vein occlusion. April 2009, p 2.

20 Anonymous: Wirksamkeit und Sicherheit von Ranibizumab unter Praxisbedingungen. Addendum. Ophthalmologe 2009;106:3.

21 Nguyen QD, Shah SM: Primary endpoint (6 months) results of ranibizumab for edema of the macula in diabetes (READ-2) study. Ophthalmology 2009;116: 2175–2181.

22 Scott IU, Edwards AR: A phase II randomized clinical trial of intravitreal bevacizumab for diabetic macular edema Ophthalmology 2007;114:1860–1867.

23 Cunningham ET, Adamis AP: Macugen Diabetic Retinopathy Study Group: A phase II randomized double masked trial of pegaptanib, an anti VEGF aptamer for diabetic macular edema. Ophthalmology 2005;112:1747–1757.
24 Quresh M, McIntosh R: Interventions for central retinal vein occlusions. An evidence-based systematic review. Ophthalmology 2007;114:507–519.
25 Luckie AP, Wroblewski JJ: A randomized prospective study of outpatient hemodilution for central retinal vein obstruction. Aust NZ J Ophthalmol 1996;24:223–232.
26 The Central Retinal Vein Occlusion Study Group Report: Evaluation of grid pattern photocoagulation for macular edema in central retinal vein occlusion: Ophthalmology 1995;102:1434–1444.
27 Ip MS, Scott IU: A randomized trial comparing the efficacy and safety of intravitreal triamcinolone with observation to treat vision loss associated with macular edema secondary to central retinal vein occlusion: the Standard Care versus Corticosteroid for Retinal Vein Occlusion (SCORE) study report 5. Arch Ophthalmol 2009;127:1101–1114.
28 http://www.clintrials.gov/ct2/show/NCT00168324/00168298.
29 Pieramici DJ, Rabena M: Ranibizumab for the treatment of macular edema associated with perfused central retinal vein occlusions. Ophthalmology 2008;115:e47–e54.
30 The Branch Vein Occlusion Study Group (BVOS): Argon laser photocoagulation for macular edema in branch vein occlusion. Am J Ophthalmol 1984;98:271–282.
31 Scott IU, Ip MS: A randomized trial comparing the efficacy and safety of intravitreal triamcinolone with standard care to treat vision loss associated with macular edema secondary to branch retinal vein occlusion: the Standard Care versus Corticosteroid for Retinal Vein Occlusion (SCORE) study report 6. Arch Ophthalmol 2009;127:1115–1128.
32 http://www.clintrials.gov/ct2/show/NCT00168324/00168298.
33 Prager F, Michels S: Intravitreal bevacizumab (Avastin) for macular edema secondary to retinal vein occlusion – twelve month results of a prospective clinical trial. Br J Ophthalmol 2009;93:452–456.
34 NHS UK – National Horizon Scanning Centre: Ranibizumab for macular oedema secondary to central or branch retinal vein occlusion. April 2009, p 3 (http://www.clintrials.gov/ct2/show/NCT00486018).
35 Jaffe GJ, Martin D: Fluocinolone acetonide implant (Retisert) for non-infectious posterior uveitis: 34 week results of a multicentre randomized clinical study. Ophthalmology 2006;113:1020–1027.
36 Williams GA, Haller JA: Dexamethasone posterior-segment drug delivery system in the treatment of macular edema resulting from uveitis or Irvine-Gass syndrome. Am J Ophthalmol 2009;147:1048–1054.
37 Cordero Coma M, Sobrin L: Intravitreal bevacizumab for treatment if uveitic macular edema. Ophthalmology 2007;114:1574–1579.
38 Arevalo F, Maia M: Intravitreal bevacizumab for refractory pseudophakic cystoids macular edema: The Pan-American Collaborative Retina Study Group. Ophthalmology 2009;116:1481–1487.

Prof. A.J. Augustin
Augenklinik
Moltkestrasse 90
DE–76133 Karlsruhe (Germany)
Tel. +49 721 9742001, Fax +49 721 9742009, E-Mail albertjaugustin@googlemail.com

Bandello F, Battaglia Parodi M (eds): Anti-VEGF.
Dev Ophthalmol. Basel, Karger, 2010, vol 46, pp 123–132

Angiogenesis and Vascular Endothelial Growth Factors in Intraocular Tumors

Guy S. Missotten[a,b] · Reinier O. Schlingemann[b] · Martine J. Jager[c]

[a]Department of Ophthalmology, Catholic University Leuven, Belgium; [b]Department of Ophthalmology, Academic Medical Center, Amsterdam, and [c]Department of Ophthalmology, Leiden University, Leiden, The Netherlands

Abstract

The role of angiogenesis in tumors appears obvious: without vessels, tumors cannot grow. However, the long-held belief that all human solid tumors are angiogenesis-dependent has been challenged by the universally disappointing results of anti-angiogenesis therapy in cancer. This may be explained by the fact that cooption of preexisting vasculature as a primary or secondary mechanism of tumor vascularization is more important than previously thought. Nevertheless, anti-angiogenesis therapy may play an important (adjuvant) role in the prevention of metastases of intraocular tumors (uveal melanoma and retinoblastoma). Antivascular endothelial growth factor therapy already plays an important role in the management of irradiation complications in tumor eyes.

The most frequent intraocular tumors are retinoblastoma in children (incidence 6–12 per million children per year) and uveal melanoma in adults (incidence 6–8 per million per year) [1]. A special characteristic of intraocular tumors is their pathway of metastasis: with the exception of massive extraocular growth or optic nerve outgrowth in retinoblastoma, metastatic dissemination is mainly hematogenous due to the absence of lymphatic vessels in the eye.

The role of angiogenesis in tumors appears obvious: without vessels, tumors cannot grow. In the 1970s, Folkman and co-workers started to work on angiogenesis, particularly in ophthalmology, which opened a large field of investigation. Folkman's hypothesis that solid tumors are angiogenesis-dependent, initiated studies of angiogenesis in tumor biology [2]. Vascular endothelial growth factor (VEGF) and many other angiogenic proteins were found to play a major role in ocular and general angiogenesis.

When a tumor starts to expand, the need for oxygen and nutrients increases. To fulfill this need, a first step can be the incorporation of existing vessels into the tumor. Secondly, the growing tumor can induce new vessel formation by stimulating sprouting from preexisting vessels (angiogenesis). However, the long-held belief that all human solid tumors are angiogenesis-dependent has been challenged by the universally disappointing results of anti-angiogenesis therapy in cancer. This may be explained by the fact that cooption of preexisting vasculature as a primary or secondary mechanism of tumor vascularization is more important than previously thought [3].

It is likely that such incorporation of choroidal vessels occurs in the early growth of uveal melanoma. Uveal melanomas are dependent on angiogenesis for growth beyond a certain size, and angiogenesis seems also necessary for metastasis. An important prognostic factor in uveal melanoma is microvascular density [4, 5], with an increased risk for metastasis in highly vascularized tumors.

A difference in vessel maturation is observed between retinoblastoma and uveal melanoma. In retinoblastoma, neovessels (vessels without differentiated pericytes as recognized by expression of α-smooth muscle actin) spread from the center of the tumor to peripheral edges, whereas in uveal melanoma, neovessels spread from the basal areas of the tumor to the tumor apex [6, 7]. As anti-angiogenic therapy targets primarily areas with a high angiogenic activity, and has less effect on established mature blood vessels, the spatial distribution of mature blood vessels in ocular tumors may influence the efficacy of anti-angiogenic therapies.

Induction of Angiogenesis in Tumors

Tumorigenesis is a multistep process involving genetic and proteomic alterations that drive the progressive transformation of cells into malignant cells, similar to an evolutionary process. One of these steps is the acquisition of angiogenic potential of primary and metastatic malignant neoplasms. Hypoxia is an important regulator of this process: many angiogenic factors are upregulated by hypoxia [8]. Furthermore, rapidly growing tumors induce cell apoptosis due to central hypoxia, and the presence of necrotic areas within large uveal melanomas have been reported as an important prognostic factor [9]. Following hypoxia, tumor cells secrete large amounts of angiogenic factors to stimulate angiogenesis. As a result, preexisting vessels become more permeable, and their endothelial cells become activated by these angiogenic factors. Out of these stimulated endothelial cells, sprouts are formed to induce new vessels. These early immature vessels are not stabilized yet, since mural cells have not been recruited. Once these new vessels undergo maturation, they become bordered by differentiated pericytes, and they become less dependent on angiogenic factors, and hence less sensitive to anti-angiogenic therapies. Vessel maturation in human retinoblastoma and uveal melanoma is very heterogenous [6], showing large variations between tumors in the numbers of neovessels.

Regulators of Angiogenesis

The role of VEGF has been investigated in uveal melanoma as well as in retinoblastoma. Expression of VEGF-A was found in retinoblastoma [10, 11], and an association between tumor volume and VEGF concentrations in ocular media was established in eyes with uveal melanoma [12–15]. Expression of VEGF receptors as well as of insulin-like growth factor receptor (IGF-1R) was found on uveal melanomas and their cell lines [16], and tumors were found to express VEGF-A, -B, -C and -D, as well as b-FGF [14, 17] (fig. 1, 2), and pigment epithelium-derived factor (PEDF) [18]. In vitro work [13] also showed that uveal melanoma cells could stimulate functions associated with angiogenesis in endothelial cells. El Filali et al. [19] recently demonstrated that when uveal melanoma cells obtained from cell lines or fresh tumor tissue were exposed to a hypoxic environment, this led to an increased VEGF production. As expanding tumors probably develop hypoxia in vivo, this may be a mechanism that stimulates angiogenesis in uveal melanomas too.

In addition, different metalloproteinases (MMPs) and matricellular proteins (SPARC, TSP1 and TSP2) [20] are expressed in uveal melanoma, while the expression of inhibitors of MMPs, the TIMPs, is decreased [21]. MMP-9 was shown to be present in 72% of uveal melanomas [22]. Canovas et al. [23] reported high levels of TIMPs in the vitreous humor of eyes containing a uveal melanoma, claiming a possible effect on tumor behavior. In retinoblastoma, a possible link between the aqueous humor and the absence of HIF-1α and NOS expression in an anterior chamber retinoblastoma was hypothesized [24].

Vascular Mimicry

Uveal melanomas and their metastases are characterized by PAS-positive patterns [25, 26]. These patterns are totally different from endothelial cell-lined blood vessels and known as 'vasculogenic mimicry' [27]. As such, angiogenesis may be not the only mechanism by which tumors acquire their microcirculation. Nine different PAS-positive patterns were described and the morphologic patterns with loops and/or networks, which probably represent nodular growth, were significantly correlated with a poor prognosis [28].

Maniotis et al. [29] showed that a vascular channel could be formed by human melanoma cells both in vitro and in vivo. This would result in non-endothelial cell-lined microcirculatory channels which are delimited only by extracellular matrix. In an animal model, transport of fluid by tumor cell-lined channels was shown [30], while in a human study, the circular sheets causing the looping patterns were shown to conduct dye and were detectable by indocyanine green dye injection and laser confocal scanning ophthalmography [31].

Fig. 1. VEGF-A protein expression in primary uveal melanoma cultures. The amount of VEGF-A protein expression measured with ELISA in supernatant of primary uveal melanoma cell cultures (cultures 1–5) under normoxic (black) and hypoxic (gray) exposure after 24 h. Expression is demonstrated in amount protein (pg/ml). 130 × 86 mm (300 × 300 dpi) [from 19].

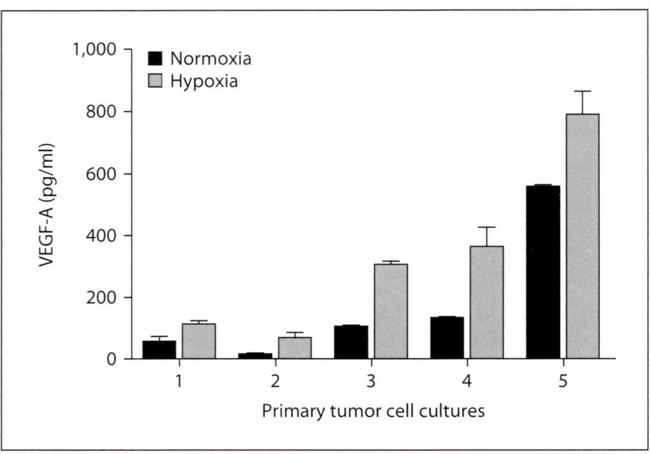

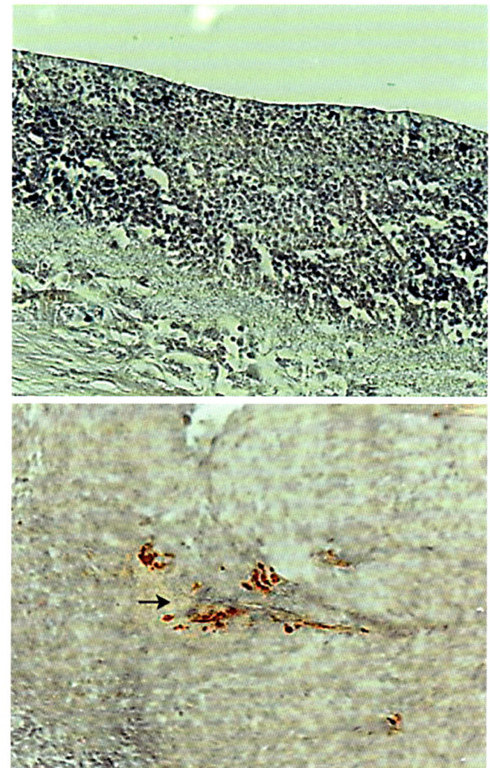

Fig. 2. Expression of VEGF-A in human uveal melanoma tissue. In situ hybridization of VEGF-A with uveal melanoma demonstrated diffuse VEGF-A expression throughout the tumors, especially around blood vessels [from 15].

Inflammation and Angiogenesis

In cancer, chronic inflammation has been demonstrated within tumor foci and a number of studies suggest that tumor-associated macrophages promote the growth, proliferation, and metastasis of neoplastic cells and can induce angiogenesis leading to tumor progression. In uveal melanoma, PAS-positive patterns were associated with endothelial cells expressing endothelial monocyte-activating polypeptide (EMAP)-II, a cytokine that attracts macrophages [32]. The presence of high numbers of macrophages carries an adverse prognosis in uveal melanoma [33]. As tumors with high numbers of infiltrating macrophages also show an increased expression of HLA class I and II and a lymphocytic infiltrate, we coined the term *inflammatory phenotype* for this category of uveal melanomas [34].

Radiation Retinopathy

Eyes that had to be removed because of complications after irradiation of uveal melanoma showed an increase in the production of VEGF in the eye, probably as a result of the tissue hypoxia caused by enhanced destruction of vascular endothelial cells in the tumor [15]. This would suggest that complications of radiation retinopathy might be susceptible to treatment with VEGF inhibitors.

Radiation retinopathy is an occlusive microangiopathy, with focal capillary closure, relative early sparing of pericytes and irregular dilation of the neighboring microvasculature [35, 36]. Eventually, capillaries as well as pericytes are lost, with resulting inner retinal non-perfusion and inner and outer retinal atrophy. Macular edema is one of the earliest signs of radiation maculopathy. Shields et al. [37] defined clinical radiation maculopathy as retinal capillary bed changes (dilation, microaneurysm, retinal hemorrhage), retinal edema, retinal exudation, nerve fiber layer infarction, or vascular sheathing affecting the area within 3 mm of the foveola. Radiation retinopathy generally occurs more than 1 year after brachytherapy. In an analysis of 1,300 patients treated with plaque radiotherapy for posterior uveal melanoma, clinical evidence of radiation maculopathy was found in 43% of patients at 5-year follow-up [38]. In a study on 125 patients, 17% had macular edema at 6 months, 40% at 12 months, 57% at 18 months and 61% at 24 months, despite treatment (transpupillary thermotherapy and laser coagulation) [39].

The size of the tumor, the radiation dose to the tumor base, and the radiation dose to the optic disk are all significant factors in the development of macular edema [39]. Depending on the size of the tumor, radiation retinopathy can be up to 25% and neovascular glaucoma may occur in 15% [40], especially after proton beam therapy for extremely large tumors [41].

Local Treatment of Radiation Retinopathy

One of the treatments of radiation retinopathy is intravitreal injection of triamcinolone, a corticosteroid. This drug had no effect on the growth of uveal melanoma cells in vitro [42]. It is currently investigated whether VEGF inhibitors have any effect on tumor cells in vitro, as different receptors and mRNA of VEGF-A isoforms are expressed in uveal melanoma cells [17, 43]. The effectiveness of the use of triamcinolone and anti-angiogenic treatments is being investigated in tumor eyes suffering from radiation retinopathy. A prospective study including 163 patients treated with three injections of periocular triamcinolone during the first year after brachytherapy showed [37] a benefit of treatment in the first 18 months after plaque radiotherapy and a significant reduction of the number of patients with poor visual acuity. Following injection of bevacizumab, 1 case of extensive cystoid macular edema showed an increase of visual acuity and decrease of central retinal optical coherence tomography thickness in the first months after the injection [44].

Treatment of Radiation-Induced Neovascular Glaucoma

Neovascular glaucoma can occur following radiation therapy of large ocular tumors. An intravitreal injection of bevacizumab (1.25 mg) can cause regression of iris and angle neovascularization within 1 week [45–47], both in iris and posterior segment melanoma, and resolution of a serous detachment within 1 month (intravitreal injection 14 months following iodine brachytherapy). Rapid regression was also seen with intravitreal injection with ranibizumab, with an improvement of rubeosis iridis 2 days after administration, and this effect lasted 6 months [48].

Metastasis and Angiogenesis

The primary site for metastases of uveal melanoma is the liver, but metastases may also occur in the lung, skin and brain. Micrometastasis of approximately 100 μm are assumed to remain dormant in the liver for many years, and are thought to become only active after angiogenesis is induced. In a murine model, metastatic uveal melanoma cells are shown to express higher VEGF levels than the primary tumor cells [49]. Nevertheless, no correlation between VEGF expression on the primary tumor and metastasis formation was found [12]. Patients with clinical metastases have higher VEGF levels in their serum compared to patients without metastases [19].

For metastasis treatment, combining various agents with different activities, including anti-angiogenic functions, may be a reasonable approach. A study combining low-dose thalidomide and interferon-α_{2b} in 6 metastatic uveal melanoma patients achieved a stabilization of metastases in the liver and lung that lasted 12 months [50].

In an animal model, low-dose angiostatin could reduce the number of hepatic micrometastases in a murine ocular melanoma model [51]. It was assumed that an alteration of VEGF expression occurred in the melanoma cells and that angiostatin inhibited migration of the melanoma cells [49]. Inhibition of VEGF in a mouse model of retinoblastoma with intravitreal bevacizumab showed a decrease in the growth of retinoblastoma in vitro and vivo [52]. Similar results were found in a murine model of uveal melanoma [53]. PEDF is an angiogenesis inhibitor that balances angiogenesis in the eye and blocks tumor progression. Although PEDF has no effect on proliferation of retinoblastoma cells in vitro, treatment with PEDF injections inhibited the growth of retinoblastoma xenografts in vivo by downregulating HIF-1α and VEGF [53]. Also, PEDF overexpression in uveal melanoma cells inhibited intraocular growth and the development of liver metastases in a murine model [53]. The use of adjuvant anecortave acetate also reduced the tumor load significantly in a retinoblastoma mouse model [54]. However, this treatment induced the development of hypoxic areas in the tumor [55]. The addition of carboplatin and also of glycolytic inhibitors had an additional treatment effect [56].

In vitro, reduction of VEGF and tumor growth was reached with RNAi targeting VEGF [57]. Nevertheless, the heterogeneity and spatial distribution of vessels, both in retinoblastoma as well as in uveal melanoma, limits anti-angiogenic treatments that only target immature vasculature. Anti-angiogenesis treatment of uveal melanoma metastases in humans has not yet been reported.

Picropodophyllin, an inhibitor of IGF-1R, was shown to block uveal melanoma growth [16]. As this drug can be given orally, clinical studies are anxiously awaited. Inhibition of ocular tumor growth was also achieved in an in vivo model by gene transduction which led to an increase in interleukin-12, a strong anti-angiogenic cytokine [58].

Treatment

The final proof of principle that cancer patients can be effectively treated with angiogenesis inhibitors is still awaited [3, 59]. Various preclinical in vitro and in vivo experiments have proven that most tumors need new vessel formation in order to grow and to form metastases, and this is also true for intraocular tumors. First of all, tumors placed in the avascular cornea do not grow until new blood vessels reach the implant. Secondly, the introduction of only one angiogenic gene can cause a switch from tumor dormancy to progressive tumor growth. Thirdly, tumor growth can be inhibited and sometimes tumor regression can be obtained just by attacking the vascular compartment with specific angiogenesis inhibitors [3].

In these model systems, angiogenesis is necessary for tumors >2 mm, and there are no indications that the same should not be true for metastases. This would say that (multiple?) metastases can form without any need for angiogenesis, especially the micrometastasis that are assumed to exist in uveal melanoma. Anti-angiogenesis may play an important role as adjuvant therapy, but a complete remediation of metastatic tumor disease based only on this mechanism seems unlikely.

After a few years of clinical experience with other malignancies, a number of considerations and questions have emerged. First, the idea of starving tumors has been called into question, because VEGF-R treatment not only starves tumors but also normalizes the highly abnormal tumor vasculature, thereby yielding the advantage of improving the delivery of cytotoxic drugs. Secondly, VEGF-R inhibitory treatment is limited by resistance/escape, and provides no definitive cure, but survival prolongation in the range of months rather than years. Also, VEGF-R inhibitors induce adverse effects because of the importance of VEGF signaling for the maintenance of quiescent endothelium in healthy organs, and probably of the neuroretina in the eye [8, 60]. Thus, anti-VEGF therapy as monotherapy of intraocular tumors or its metastases will not be an option, and novel strategies focusing on combination treatments are needed.

References

1 Egan KM, Seddon JM, Glynn RJ, Gragoudas ES, Albert DM: Epidemiologic aspects of uveal melanoma. Surv Ophthalmol 1988;32:239–251.

2 Folkman J: Tumour angiogenesis: therapeutic implications. N Engl J Med 1971;285:1182–1186.

3 Verheul HM, Voest EE, Schlingemann RO: Are tumours angiogenesis-dependent? J Pathol 2004; 202:5–13.

4 Foss AJ, Alexander RA, Jefferies LW, Hungerford JL, Harris AL, Lightman S: Microvessel count predicts survival in uveal melanoma. Cancer Res 1996;56: 2900–2903.

5 Makitie T, Summanen P, Tarkkanen A, Kivela T: Microvascular density in predicting survival of patients with choroidal and ciliary body melanoma. Invest Ophthalmol Vis Sci 1999;40:2471–2480.

6 Pina Y, Boutrid H, Schefler A, Dubovy S, Feuer W, Jockovich ME, Murray TG: Blood vessel maturation in retinoblastoma tumors: spatial distribution of neovessels and mature vessels and its impact on ocular treatment. Invest Ophthalmol Vis Sci 2009; 50:1020–1024.

7 Pina Y, Cebulla CM, Murray TG, Alegret A, Dubovy SR, Boutrid H, Feuer W, Mutapcic L, Jockovich ME: Blood vessel maturation in human uveal melanoma: spatial distribution of neovessels and mature vasculature. Ophthalmic Res 2009;41:160–169.

8 Witmer AN, Vrensen GF, van Noorden CJ, Schlingemann RO: Vascular endothelial growth factors and angiogenesis in eye disease. Prog Retin Eye Res 2003;22:1–29.

9 Missotten GS: Doctoral Thesis. Angiogenesis and Screening in Uveal Melanoma. Leiden, The Netherlands, 2005.

10 Kvanta A, Steen B, Seregard S: Expression of VEGF in retinoblastoma but not in posterior uveal melanoma. Exp Eye Res 1996;63:511–518.

11 Stitt AW, Simpson DA, Boocock C, Gardiner TA, Murphy GM, Archer DB: Expression of VEGF and its receptors is regulated in eyes with intraocular tumours. J Pathol 1998;186:306–312.

12 Sheidow TG, Hooper PL, Crukley C, Young J, Heathcote JG: Expression of VEGF in uveal melanoma and its correlation with metastasis. Br J Ophthalmol 2000;84:750–756.

13 Boyd SR, Tan D, Bruce C, Gittos A, Neale MH, Hungerford JL, Charnock-Jones S, Cree IA: Vascular endothelial growth factor is elevated in ocular fluids of eyes harbouring uveal melanoma: identification of a potential therapeutic window. Br J Ophthalmol 2002;86:448–452.

14 Boyd SR, Tan DS, de Souza L, Neale MH, Myatt NE, Alexander RA, Robb M, Hungerford JL, Cree IA: Uveal melanomas express vascular endothelial growth factor and basic fibroblast growth factor and support endothelial cell growth. Br J Ophthalmol 2002;86:440–447.

15 Missotten GS, Notting IC, Schlingemann RO, Zijlmans HJ, Lau C, Eilers PH, Keunen JE, Jager MJ: Vascular endothelial growth factor-A in eyes with uveal melanoma. Arch Ophthalmol 2006;124:1428–1434.

16 Economou MA, Andersson S, Vasilcanu D, All-Ericsson C, Menu E, Girnita A, Girnita L, Axelson M, Seregard S, Larsson O: Oral picropodophyllin is well tolerated in vivo and inhibits IGF-1R expression and growth of uveal melanoma. Invest Ophthalmol Vis Sci 2008;49:2337–2342.

17 Notting IC, Missotten GS, Sijmons B, Boonman ZF, Keunen JE, van der Pluijm G: Angiogenesic profile of uveal melanoma. Curr Eye Res 2006;31:775–785.

18 Yang H, Cheng R, Liu G, Zhong Q, Li C, Cai W, Yang Z, Ma J, Yang X, Gao G: PEDF inhibits growth of retinoblastoma by anti-angiogenic activity. Cancer Sci 2009;100:2419–2425.

19 El Filali M, Missotten GS, Maat W, Ly LV, Luyten GPM, van der Velden PA, Jager MJ: Invest Ophthalmol Vis Sci 2010;51:2329–2337.

20 Ordonez JL, Paraoan L, Hiscott P, Gray D, Garcia-Finana M, Grierson I, Damato B: Differential expression of angioregulatory matricellular proteins in posterior uveal melanoma. Melanoma Res 2005;15: 495–502.

21 Van der Velden PA, Zuidervaart W, Hurks MH, Pavey S, Ksander BR, Krijgsman E, Frants RR, Tensen CP, Willemze R, Jager MJ, Gruis NA: Expression profiling reveals that methylation of TIMP-3 is involved in uveal melanoma development. Int J Cancer 2003;106:472–479.

22 Sahin A, Kiratli H, Tezel GG, Soylemezoglu F, Bilgic S: Expression of vascular endothelial growth factor A, matrix metalloproteinase-9 and extravascular matrix patterns in iris and ciliary body melanomas. Ophthalmic Res 2007;39:40–44.

23 Canovas D, Rennie IG, Nichols CE, Sisley K: Local environmental influences on uveal melanoma. Vitreous humor promotes uveal melanoma invasion, whereas the aqueous can be inhibitory. Cancer 2008;112:1787–1794.

24 Crosby MB, Hubbard GB, Gallie BL, Grossniklaus HE: Anterior diffuse retinoblastoma: mutational analysis and immunofluorescence staining. Arch Pathol Lab Med 2009;133:1215–1218.

25 Rummelt V, Mehaffey MG, Campbell RJ, Pe'er J, Bentler SE, Woolson RF, Naumann GO, Folberg R: Microcirculation architecture of metastases from primary ciliary body and choroidal melanomas. Am J Ophthalmol 1998;126:303–305.

26 Folberg R, Rummelt V, Parys-van Ginderdeuren R, Hwang T, Woolson RF, Pe'er J, Gruman LM: The prognostic value of tumour blood vessel morphology in primary uveal melanoma. Ophthalmology 1993;100:1389–1398.

27 Bhat P, Jakobiec FA, Folberg R: Comparison of tumor-associated vasculatures in uveal and cutaneous melanomas. Semin Ophthalmol 2009;24:166–171.

28 Makitie T, Summanen P, Tarkkanen A, Kivela T: Microvascular loops and networks as prognostic indicators in choroidal and ciliary body melanomas. J Natl Cancer Inst 1999;91:359–367.

29 Maniotis AJ, Folberg R, Hess A, Seftor EA, Gardner LMG, Pe'er J, Trent JM, Meltzer PS, Hendrix MJC: Vascular channel formation by human melanoma cells in vivo and in vitro; vascular mimicry. Am J Pathol 1999;155:739–752.

30 Clarijs R, Otte-Holler I, Ruiter DJ, de Waal RMW: Presence of a fluid-conducting meshwork in xenografted cutaneous and primary human uveal melanoma. Invest Ophthalmol Vis Sci 2002;43:912–918.

31 Shields CL, Shields JA, De Potter P: Patterns of indocyanine green videoangiography of choroidal tumors. Br J Ophthalmol 1995;79:237–245.

32 Clarijs R, Schalkwijk L, Ruiter DJ, de Waal RM: EMAP-II expression is associated with macrophage accumulation in primary uveal melanoma. Invest Ophthalmol Vis Sci 2003;44:1801–1806.

33 Makitie T, Summanen P, Tarkkanen A, Kivela T: Tumor-infiltrating macrophages (CD68+ cells) and prognosis in malignant uveal melanoma. Invest Ophthalmol Vis Sci 2001;42:1414–1421.

34 Maat W, Ly LV, Jordanova ES, de Wolff-Rouendaal D, Schalij-Delfos NE, Jager MJ: Monosomy of chromosome 3 and an inflammatory phenotype occur together in uveal melanoma. Invest Ophthalmol Vis Sci 2008;49:505–510.

35 Archer DB: Doyne Lecture. Responses of retinal and choroidal vessels to ionizing radiation. Eye 1993;7:1–13.

36 Irvine AR, Woor IS: Radiation retinopathy as an experimental model for ischemic proliferative retinopathy and rubeosis iridis. Am J Ophthalmol 1987; 103:790–797.

37 Horgan N, Shields CL, Mashayekhi A, Salazar PF, Materin MA, O'Reagan M, Shields JA: Periocular triamcinolone for prevention of macular edema after plaque radiotherapy of uveal melanoma: a randomized controlled trial. Arch Ophthalmol 2009; 116:1383–1390.

38 Gunduz K, Shields CL, Shileds JA, Cater J, Freire JE, Brady LW: Radiation retinopathy following plaque radiotherapy for posterior uveal melanoma. Arch Ophthalmol 1999;117:609–614.

39 Horgan N, Shields CL, Mashayekhi A, Teixeira LF, Materin MA, Shields JA: Early macular morphological changes following plaque radiotherapy for uveal melanoma. Retina 2008;28:263–273.

40 Krema H, Simpson ER, Pavlin CJ, Payne D, Vasquez LM, McGowan H: Management of ciliary body melanoma with iodine-125 plaque therapy. Can J Ophthalmol 2009;44:395–400.

41 Boyd SR, Gittos A, Richter M, Hungerford JL, Errington RD, Cree IA: Proton beam therapy and iris neovascularisation in uveal melanoma. Eye 2006;20:832–836.
42 El Filali M, Homminga I, Maat W, Van der Velden PA, Jager MJ: Triamcinolone acetonide and anecortave acetate do not stimulate uveal melanoma cell growth. Mol Vis 2008;14:1752–1759.
43 Ijland SA, Jager MJ, Heijdra BM, Westphal JR, Peek R: Expression of angiogenic and immunosuppressive factors by uveal melanoma cell Lines. Melanoma Res 1999;9:445–450.
44 Ziemssen F, Voelker M, Altpeter E, Bartz-Schmidt KU, Gelisken F: Intravitreal bevacizumab treatment of radiation maculopathy due to brachytherapy in choroidal melanoma. Acta Ophthalmol 2007;85: 579–580.
45 Jaissle GB, Ulmer A, Henke-Fahle S, Fierlbeck G, Bartz-Schmidt KU, Szurman P: Suppression of melanoma-associated neoangiogenesis by bevacizumab. Arch Dermatol 2008;144:525–527.
46 Bianciotto C, Shields CL, Kang B, Shields JA: Treatment of iris melanoma and secondary neovascular glaucoma using bevacizumab and plaque radiotherapy. Arch Ophthalmol 2008;126:578–579.
47 Vásquez LM, Somani S, Altomare F, Simpson ER: Intracameral bevacizumab in the treatment of neovascular glaucoma and exudative retinal detachment after brachytherapy in choroidal melanoma. Can J Ophthalmol 2009;44:106–107.
48 Dunavoelgyi R, Zehetmayer M, Simader C, Schmidt-Erfurth U: Rapid improvement of radiation-induced neovascular glaucoma and exudative retinal detachment after a single intravitreal ranibizumab injection. Clin Exp Ophthalmol 2007;35:878–880.
49 Yang H, Xu Z, Luvone PM, Grossniklaus HE: Angiostatin decreases cell migration and VEGF to PEDF RNA ratio in vitro and in a murine ocular melanoma model. Mol Vis 2006;12:511–517.
50 Solti M, Berd D, Mastrangelo MJ, Sato T: A pilot study of low-dose thalidomide and interferon-α_{2b} in patients with metastatic melanoma who failed prior treatment. Melanoma Res 2007;17:225–231.
51 Yang H, Akor C, Dithmar S, Grossniklaus HE: Low-dose adjuvant angiostatin decreases hepatic micrometastasis in murine ocular melanoma model. Mol Vis 2004;10:987–995.
52 Lee SY, Kim DK, Cho JH, Koh JY, Yoon YH: Inhibitory effect of bevacizumab on the angiogenesis and growth of retinoblastoma. Arch Ophthalmol 2008;126:953–958.
53 Yang H, Grossniklaus HE: Constitutive overexpression of pigment epithelium-derived factor inhibits ocular melanoma growth and metastasis. Invest Ophthalmol Vis Sci 2010;51:28–34.
54 Jockovich M, Murray TG, Escalona-Benz E, Hernandez E, Feuer W: Anecortave acetate as single and adjuvant therapy in the treatment of retinal tumors of $LH_{BETA}T_{AG}$ mice. Invest Ophthalmol Vis Sci 2006;47:1264–1268.
55 Boutrid H, Pina Y, Cebulla CM, Feuer WJ, Lampidis TJ, Jockovich ME, Murray TG: Invest Ophthalmol Vis Sci 2009;50:5537–5543.
56 Boutrid H, Jockovich ME, Murray TG, Pina Y, Feuer WJ, Lampidis TJ, Cebulla CM: Targeting hypoxia, a novel treatment for advanced retinoblastoma. Invest Ophthalmol Vis Sci 2008;49:2799–2805.
57 Jia RB, Zhang YX, Zhou YX, Song X, Liu HY, Wang LZ, Luo M, Lu J, Ge SF, Fan XQ: VEGF-targeted RNA interference suppresses angiogenesis and tumor growth of retinoblastoma. Ophthalmic Res 2007;32:108–115.
58 Albini A, Fassini G, Nicolo M, Dell'Eva R, Vene R, Cammarota R, Barberis M, Noonan DM: Inhibition of a vascular ocular tumor growth by IL-12 gene transfer. Clin Exp Metastasis 2007;24:485–493.
59 Jager MJ: Angiogenesis in uveal melanoma. Ophthalmic Res 2006;38:248–250.
60 Saint-Geniez M, Maharaj AS, Walshe TE, Tucker BA, Sekiyama E, Kurihara T, Darland DC, Young MJ, D'Amore PA: Endogenous VEGF is required for visual function: evidence for a survival role on Müller cells and photoreceptors. PLoS One 2008;3: e3554.

Guy S. Missotten
Department Ophthalmology, Academic Medical Center
Meibergdreef 9, Post Box 22660
NL–1100DD Amsterdam (The Netherlands)
Tel. +31 20 566 5907, Fax +31 20 566 9078, E-Mail guy.missotten@uzleuven.be

Bandello F, Battaglia Parodi M (eds): Anti-VEGF.
Dev Ophthalmol. Basel, Karger, 2010, vol 46, pp 133–139

Antivascular Endothelial Growth Factors in Anterior Segment Diseases

Stefan Scholl · Janna Kirchhof · Albert J. Augustin

Augenklinik, Karlsruhe, Germany

Abstract

Proangiogenic growth factors, mainly VEGF (vascular endothelial growth factor) play a significant role in anterior segment diseases, characterized by neovascularization. Newly grown vessels in the cornea can lead to an impairment of transparency and visual acuity. Neovascularization of the iris (rubeosis iridis) and the anterior chamber angle are caused by ischemic retinopathies, usually leading to neovascular glaucoma with serious loss of vision. A pterygium is characterized, amongst others, by fibrovascular proliferation and may have vision threatening consequences if left untreated. Several antiangiogenic drugs have evolved in the last decade, mainly used for the treatment of choroidal neovascularization in age-related macular degeneration. Bevacizumab though, is also widely used off-label, in topic form or as an intracameral injection, to treat anterior segment neovascularization with encouraging results.

Antivascular Endothelial Growth Factor in Corneal Neovascularization

Under physiologic conditions the cornea has the unique feature of being avascular, actively maintained by expression of antiangiogenic and antilymphangiogenic factors. Under pathologic conditions, vessels invade the cornea form the limbal vascular plexus. Corneal neovascularization (NV) is a final pathway common to numerous ocular insults and disorders such as infection, inflammation, ischemia, degeneration, loss of the limbal stem cell barrier and trauma. The result is an impairment in corneal transparency and visual acuity. Occasionally, the newly grown vessels can serve a beneficial role in clearing infections, wound healing and arresting stromal melts. The disadvantages overweigh though. Corneal NV often causes tissue scarring, corneal edema, lipid deposition and persistent inflammation. Corneal NV has been reported in about 4% of patients presenting for general ophthalmologic care in the USA, representing an estimated 1.4 million individuals [1]. About 12% of these cases are associated with an impairment in visual acuity [1]. The most common causes of corneal infectious blindnesses in the Western world (herpetic keratitis) and the developing countries (trachoma) are accompanied by corneal NV.

An extended wearing of soft contact lenses is another major cause of corneal NV. It is estimated that about 125,000–470,000 people in the USA wearing soft contact lenses show a certain degree of corneal NV [1].

An impaired visual acuity is not the only negative result of newly grown corneal vessels. Corneal NV leads to the loss of the immune privilege of the cornea. The result is a worsening of the prognosis of penetrating keratoplasty being a major cause for corneal graft rejection. On the other hand, various risk factors have been shown to be associated with an increased likelihood of corneal NV after penetrating keratoplasty [2].

Currently, topical steroids remain the first-choice therapy, because corneal NV is assumed to be secondary to some degree of inflammation. Well-known side effects include cataract, glaucoma and the increased risk for infections. When inflammation is not the cause, such as in diseases associated with deficiency of limbal cells or corneal hypoxia, anti-inflammatory corticosteroids have little or no effect on the growth of the vessels. Other therapeutic options include topical non-steroidal anti-inflammatory agents, laser photocoagulation, fine-needle diathermy, photodynamic therapy and restoration of the ocular surface with the use of conjunctival, limbal or amniotic membrane transplantation. The treatment is often ineffective or vessel recanalization occurs, requiring multiple treatment sessions.

The rapid progress in angiogenesis research in the last few years has led to the development of several novel, specific antiangiogenic drugs for use in both oncology and ophthalmology. A major focus of the research into antiangiogenic therapy is vascular endothelial growth factor (VEGF), which is known to promote several steps in angiogenesis, including proteolytic activities, endothelial cell proliferation, endothelial cell migration and capillary tube formation [3]. Its essential role in normal embryogenic vasculogenesis and angiogenesis was supported by findings that inactivation of a single VEGF allele in mice resulted in death of the embryo. VEGF is both necessary and sufficient for the occurrence of pathologic ocular NV in multiple ocular tissues. It is thought to be a key mediator in the development of corneal NV. VEGF is upregulated in inflamed and vascularized corneas. Corneal epithelial and endothelial cells, vascular endothelial cells of limbal vessels, fibroblasts and macrophages in scar tissue have all been found to excrete VEGF. The concentration of VEGF molecules and receptors is considerably higher in diseased corneas than in normal or avascular abnormal corneas. VEGF exerts its activity by binding to several high-affinity transmembrane endothelial cell receptors, especially VEGFR-1 (Flt-1) and VEGFR-2 (KDR/Flk-1). This leads to intracellular receptor phosphorylation, which in turn triggers the relevant intracellular downstream receptor pathways [4].

VEGF inhibitors, such as pegaptanib (Macugen®), ranibizumab (Lucentis®) and bevacizumab (Avastin®) are currently used for the treatment of neovascular age-related macular degeneration. The first two drugs have been approved by the US Food and Drug Administration for use in wet AMD.

Bevacizumab has been approved for use in oncology, but is also widely used on an off-label basis to treat macular edema resulting from retinal vein occlusion (RVO), proliferative diabetic retinopathy (PDR) and to treat corneal NV. Bevacizumab is a full-length recombinant humanized monoclonal antibody that binds to and inhibits the biological activity of all five human VEGF-A isoforms (VEGF-115, -121, -165, -189, -206). It prevents VEGF-A from ligating to its endothelial receptors, but does not influence other members of the VEGF gene family. Following reports that the systemic application of bevacizumab in animal models inhibited inflammatory corneal NV [5, 6], bevacizumab could have been shown to be safe and efficient in reducing corneal NV without local or systemic side effects [7, 8], administered topically as eyedrops [9–11] and subconjunctivally [12–14]. It has also been suggested that it might be used as pretransplantation treatment in penetrating keratoplasty [15]. Many aspects of topically administered bevacizumab though, including the optimal dosing for modulating the neovascular process, the long-term safety and long-term stability of treatment results, are not well known yet with only a few studies existing.

Anti-VEGF in the Treatment of Rubeosis Iridis

Neovascular glaucoma (NVG) is a potentially devastating glaucoma, where delayed diagnosis or poor management can result in complete loss of vision or, quite possibly, loss of the globe itself. Early diagnosis of the disease, followed by immediate treatment, is imperative. Retinal ischemia is the most common and important mechanism in most, if not all, cases that result in the anterior segment changes causing NVG. Ischemic retinopathies such as PDR and RVO can cause new vessel growth on the iris (rubeosis iridis, iris rubeosis, iris NV) and in the anterior chamber angle that can lead to NVG with serious consequences for the patients. RVO is the most common retinal vascular disease after diabetic retinopathy with a cumulative 10-year incidence of 1.6% [16]. Central retinal artery occlusion can also cause NV of the iris and NVG as a result of ocular ischemia, with an incidence of 1–20% [17–19].

The disease management usually attempts to control the ocular ischemia, aiming for a regression of the iris rubeosis. Panretinal photocoagulation (PRP) is the only routine treatment of choice. However, PRP often takes several weeks to induce neovascular regression. During this period, progressive angle closure and optic nerve damage may occur as a result of the elevated intra-ocular pressure [20]. VEGF levels are indirectly reduced after PRP in patients with ischemic retinal disorders [21]. However, PRP alone is not successful in halting iris NV in every patient, especially those with severe and rapid neovascular progression [22].

VEGF is an important regulator of pathological NV of the iris (rubeosis iridis, iris rubeosis, iris NV) in patients with NVG secondary to proliferative vasculopathies. The concentration of VEGF is elevated in the aqueous humor of these patients and is up to 40- to 113-fold higher in patients with NVG compared to patients with open angle glaucoma or cataract. In addition to VEGF, basic fibroblast growth factor, platelet-derived growth factor and insulin like growth factor have a role in the development of iris NV (rubeosis). Nevertheless, direct targeting of VEGF might be a possible therapeutic strategy to treat NV. The reduced neovascular activity may lead to a decreased release of inflammatory cytokines from the iris.

Intracameral injection of bevacizumab is currently tested in clinical trials. It has been shown that intracameral injection of bevacizumab reduces the aqueous humor level of VEGF and the iris NV itself. A marked regression of anterior segment NV and relief of symptoms could be observed as early as 48 h after the intracameral injection of the drug. A complete remission of the iris NV could be observed within 3 weeks after the injection [23]. In some cases, recurrent leakage was seen as early as 4 weeks necessitating repeat injection [23].

The aqueous humor concentration of VEGF has been shown to be reduced by about 10- to 30-fold 1 week after the treatment [24, 25]. Intracameral bevacizumab has no harmful effects on corneal endothelium. No significant progression in polymegatism and pleomorphism of corneal endothelial cells could be observed [25].

Several case reports and case series exist proving the short-term efficacy of intracameral bevacizumab in iris NV. In 2007, Raghuram et al. [26] have shown that intracameral injection of bevacizumab helped in the successful regression of an anterior chamber neovascular membrane in a painful blind eye with the effect being persistent even after 6 months of follow-up.

With the positive effect of intracameral bevacizumab as monotherapy proven, the effects of a combination therapy have been studied. Patients with rubeotic glaucoma secondary to ischemic central RVO were treated with intracameral bevacizumab in order to affect the outcome of their disease. In addition, the patients underwent episodes of cycloablative and panretinal laser treatment. They were followed for more than 6 months and achieved some stability with a combination of these modalities [27]. Despite these encouraging results, larger studies are needed to prove the long-term efficacy and safety of intracameral bevacizumab for iris rubeosis.

Anti-VEGF in the Treatment of Pterygium

A pterygium (Greek word 'ptery' meaning 'wing') is a very common degenerative condition of the conjunctiva, usually appearing in the form of a triangular growth of conjunctival fibrovascular tissue on the corneal surface. Although the exact cause of this lesion is not completely understood, it is associated with numerous risk factors such as infrared and ultraviolet radiation, trauma and topical irritations. A pterygium can have vision threatening consequences if left untreated.

Histopathologically a pterygium is characterized by elastotic degeneration of collagen and fibrovascular proliferation. It is suggested that an initial disruption of the limbal corneal-conjunctival barrier is followed by a progressive active 'conjunctivalization' of the cornea in which cellular proliferation, inflammation and angiogenesis are implicated. Recently the role of this inflammation and fibrovascular proliferation has been particularly highlighted as important factors in the pathogenesis of pterygia. Many growth factors, amongst them VEGF, chemically stimulate angiogenesis and have been observed in fibroblastic and inflammatory pterygium cells. It has been suggested that not only an overexpression of VEGF, but also the absence of angiogenesis inhibitors play a decisive role in the pathogenesis of pterygia [28].

The treatment options include medical and surgical approaches. The administration of artificial tears as well as steroids or non-steroidal anti-inflammatory agents can reduce the inflammatory response and relieve the symptoms. Despite a wide variety of surgical techniques and adjunct drugs (5-fluorouracil, mitomycin C) the recurrence rates show high variations from 50–80% for the simple excision to 5–15% for the more advanced techniques [29, 30].

The overexpression of VEGF in pterygium tissue led to the hypothesis that the application (subconjunctival or topical) of an anti-VEGF agent could induce regression when used at early stages or prevent recurrence when used as an adjunct to pterygium surgery or/and at the early stages of recurrent pterygium. Bahar et al. [30] have shown that a single subconjunctival injection of bevacizumab at the limbus had no effect on new vessel formation in recurrent pterygium.

A case series [31] proved that a single subconjunctival application of ranibizumab in 1 case and bevacizumab in 2 cases was effective in causing regression of conjunctival microvessels in inflamed or residual pterygia. Although hopes could be raised, a randomized prospective clinical study [32] conducted in 30 patients suggested that the single use of 1.25 mg bevacizumab did not affect the recurrence rate or early postoperative conjunctival erythema or healing of the cornea following pterygium excision. Another study [33] has shown that bevacizumab was not effective in preventing a recurrence after pterygium excision. Bevacizumab has been proven to completely prevent the recurrence in only a few cases [34]. In most cases the anti-VEGF drug could only delay the recurrence of the pterygium [35].

Currently the data in the administration of subconjunctival or topical anti-VEGF drugs for the treatment of pterygia are not conclusive. More controlled prospective randomized clinical studies incorporating a large number of patients and long-term follow-up would be necessary to better understand and to investigate the different treatment strategies, the dosage needed as well as the route of application.

References

1 Lee P, Wang CC, Adamis AP: Ocular neovascularization: an epidemiologic review. Surv Ophthalmol 1998;43:245–269.

2 Dana MR, Strellein JW: Loss and restoration of immune privilege in eyes with corneal neovascularization. Invest Ophthalmol Vis Sci 1996;37:2485–2494.

3 Chang JH, Gabison EE, Kato T, et al: Corneal neovascularization. Curr Opin Ophthalmol 2001;12: 242–249.

4 Penn JS, Madan A, Caldwell RB, et al: Vascular endothelial growth factor in eye disease. Prog Retin Eye Res 2008;27:331–371.

5 Manzano RP, Peyman GA, Khan P, et al: Inhibition of experimental corneal neovascularization by bevacizumab (Avastin). Br J Ophthalmol 2007;91:804–807.

6 Bock F, Onderka J, Rummelt C, et al: Safety profile of topical VEGF neutralization at the cornea. Invest Ophthalmol Vis Sci 2009;50:2095–2102.

7 Dastjerdi MH, Al-Arfaj KM, Nallasamy N, et al: Topical bevacizumab in the treatment of corneal neovascularization: results of a prospective, open label, noncomparative study. Arch Ophthalmol 2009;127:381–389.

8 Jacobs DS, Lim M, Carrasquillo KG, et al: Bevacizumab for corneal neovascularization. Ophthalmology 2009;116:592–593.

9 De Stafeno JJ, Kim T: Topical bevacizumab therapy for corneal neovascularization. Arch Ophthalmol 2007;125:834–836.

10 Kim SW, Ha BJ, Kim EK, et al: The effect of topical bevacizumab on corneal neovascularization. Ophthalmology 2008;115:e33–e38.

11 Uy HS, Chan PS, Ang RE: Topical bevacizumab and ocular surface neovascularization in patients with Stevens-Johnson syndrome. Cornea 2008;27:70–73.

12 Erdurmus M, Totan Y: Subconjunctival bevacizumab for corneal neovascularization. Graefes Arch Clin Exp Ophthalmol 2007;245:1577–1579.

13 Doctor PP, Bhat PV, Foster CS: Subconjunctival bevacizumab for corneal neovascularization. Cornea 2008;27:992–995.

14 Bahar I, Kaiserman I, McAllum P, et al: Subconjunctival bevacizumab injection for corneal neovascularization in recurrent pterygium. Curr Eye Res 2008;33:23–28.

15 Mackenzie SE, Tucker WR, Poole TR: Bevacizumab (Avastin) for corneal neovascularization-corneal light shield soaked application. Cornea 2009;28:246–247.

16 Wand M, Dueker DK, Aiello LM, et al: Effects of panretinal photocoagulation on rubeosis iridis, angle neovascularization and neovascular glaucoma. Am J Ophthalmol 1978;86:332–339.

17 Gartner S, Henkind P: Neovascularization of the iris (rubeosis iridis). Surv Ophthalmol 1978;22:291–312.

18 Duker JS, Brown GC: Neovascularization of the optic nerve associated with obstruction of the central retinal artery. Ophthalmology 1989;96:87–91.

19 Hayreh SS, Podhajsky P: Ocular neovascularization with retinal vascular occlusion. II. Occurrence in central and branch retinal artery occlusion. Arch Ophthalmol 1982;100:1585–1596.

20 Ehlers JP, Spirn MJ, Lam A, et al: Comparison intravitreal bevacizumab/panretinal photocoagulation versus panretinal photocoagulation alone in the treatment of neovascular glaucoma. Retina 2008;28: 696–702.

21 Tripathi RC, Li J, Tripathi BJ, et al: Increased level of vascular endothelial growth factor in aqueous humor of patients with neovascular glaucoma. Ophthalmology 1998;105:232–237.

22 Sivak-Callcott JA, O'Day DM, Gass JD, Tsai JC: Evidence-based recommendations for the diagnosis and treatment of neovascular glaucoma. Ophthalmology 2001;108:1767–1776.

23 Chalam KV, Guphta SK, Grover S, et al: Intracameral Avastin dramatically resolves iris neovascularization and reverses neovascular glaucoma. Eur J Ophthalmol 2008;18:255–262.

24 Sawada O, Kawamura H, Kakinoki M, et al: Vascular endothelial growth factor in aqueous humor before and after intravitreal injection of bevacizumab in eyes with diabetic retinopathy. Arch Ophthalmol 2007;125:1363–1366.

25 Lim TH, Bae SH, Cho YJ, et al: Concentration of vascular endothelial growth factor after intracameral bevacizumab injection in eyes with neovascular glaucoma. Korean J Ophthalmol 2009;23:188–192.

26 Raghuram A, Saravanan VR, Narendran V: Intracameral injection of bevacizumab (Avastin) to treat anterior chamber neovascular membrane in a painful blind eye. Indian J Ophthalmol 2007;55:460–462.

27 Qureshi K, Kashani S, Kelly SP: Intracameral bevacizumab for rubeotic glaucoma secondary to retinal vein occlusion. Int Ophthalmol 2009;29:537–539.

28 Mauro J, Foster CS: Pterygia: pathogenesis and the role of subconjunctival bevacizumab in treatment. Semin Ophthalmol 2009;24:130–134.

29 Fisher JP: Pterygium: follow-up. Updated January 12, 2009. http://emedicine.nedscape.com/article/1192527-followup.

30 Bahar I, Kaiserman I, Weisbrod M, et al: Extensive versus limited pterygium excision with conjunctival autograft: outcomes and recurrence rates. Curr Eye Res 2008;33:435–440.
31 Mansour AM: Treatment of inflamed pterygia or residual pterygial bed. Br J Ophthalmol 2009;93:864–865.
32 Razeghinejad MR, Hosseini H, Ahmadi F, et al: Preliminary results of subconjunctival bevacizumab in primary pterygium excision. Ophthalmic Res 2009;43:134–138.
33 Leippi S, Grehn F, Geerling G: Antiangiogenic therapy for pterigium recurrence (in German). Ophthalmologe 2009;106:413–419.
34 Wu PC, Kuo HK, Tai MH, et al: Topical bevacizumab eyedrops for limbal-conjunctival neovascularization in impending recurrent pterygium. Cornea 2009;28:103–104.
35 Fallah MR, Khosravi K, Hashemian MN, et al: Efficacy of topical bevacizumab for inhibiting growth of impending recurrent pterygium. Curr Eye Res 2010;35:17–22.

Prof. A.J. Augustin
Augenklinik
Moltkestrasse 90
DE–76133 Karlsruhe (Germany)
Tel. +49 721 9742001, Fax +49 721 9742009, E-Mail albertjaugustin@googlemail.com

Author Index

Subject Index